MW00884811

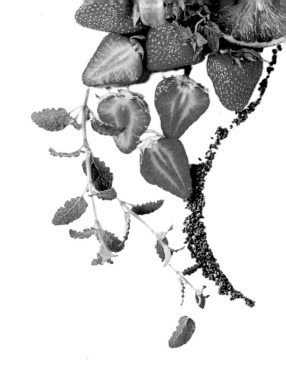

FOUNDATIONS
OF
NUTRITION

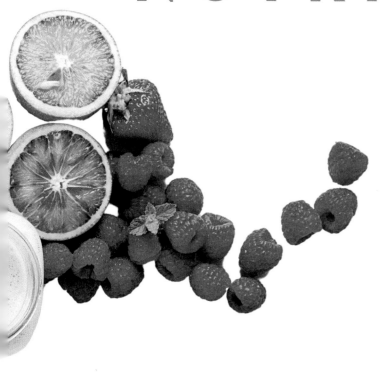

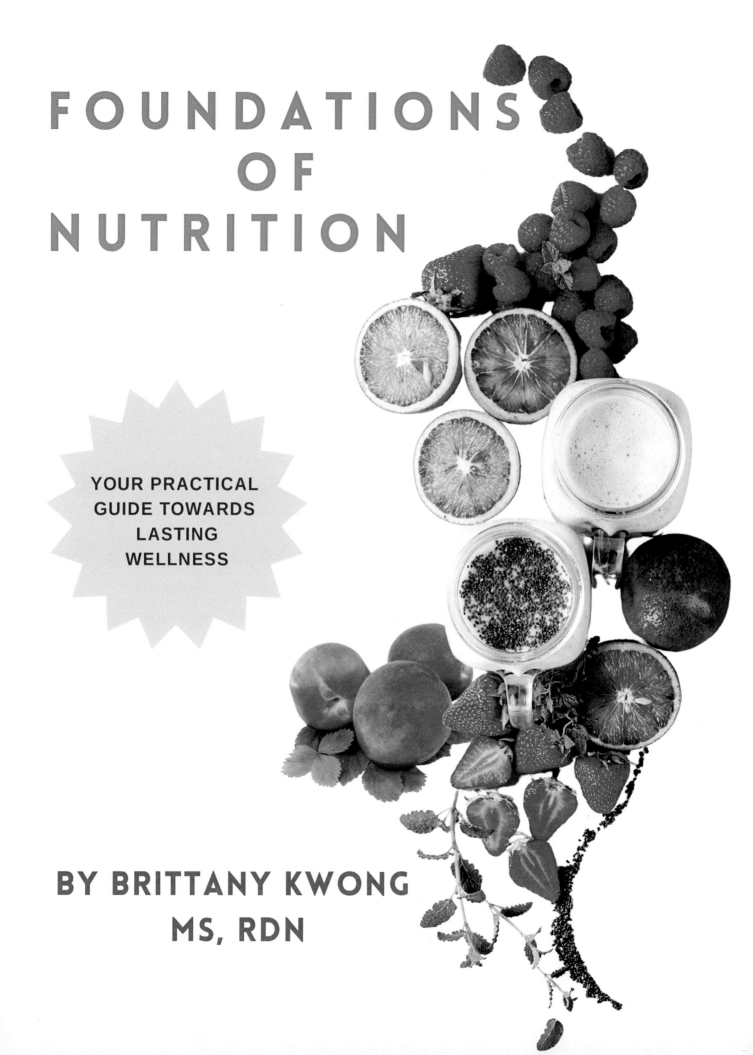

FOUNDATIONS OF NUTRITION

YOUR PRACTICAL GUIDE TOWARDS LASTING WELLNESS

BY BRITTANY KWONG
MS, RDN

Acknowledgments

My heartfelt gratitude extends to my friends and family for their unwavering support and encouragement throughout this journey. A special thank you to my mom, dad, and brother for their lifelong guidance, encouragement, and love. You have been my constant pillars of strength.

Deep appreciation and gratefulness to my Aunt Sue, Jerrin, Alex, and Janet for their invaluable time and effort in reading and editing this book. Your insights and suggestions were instrumental in bringing this project to fruition.

None of this would have been possible without the incredible people listed here, and of course, many more who have contributed in countless ways. Thank you all for being an integral part of this journey.

This book is dedicated to my parents, who have always been there for me. Your perseverance and dedication are the foundation of my success, and I aspire to embody those same qualities in my own life. Thank you for everything.

Brittany Kwong

your healthnut

FOUNDATIONS OF NUTRITION

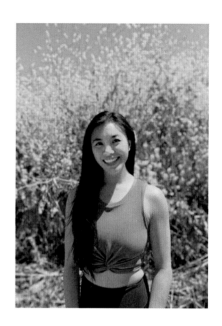

Welcome to the Foundations of Nutrition Guide: your practical guide towards lasting wellness!

Hello! My name is Brittany Kwong and I am a registered dietitian nutritionist on a mission to empower people through holistic wellness. I hold a Master of Science degree in Nutrition, Healthspan, and Longevity from the University of Southern California, where I had the privilege of studying under the guidance of Dr. Valter Longo, a pioneer in longevity research. This educational journey has fueled my commitment to sharing evidence-based nutritional practices that go beyond fleeting trends while fostering long-term well-being.

Embarking on a journey toward a healthier lifestyle doesn't have to be overwhelming. In an era saturated with conflicting nutritional information, this guide serves as your compass. Let's carve out a few moments together to lay the groundwork for a healthier, more energized version of you.

So why this guide?

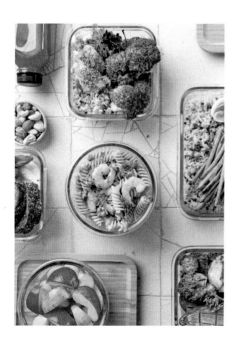

Life gets crazy and finding the time to prioritize your health can feel like an impossible task. That's where this guide comes in. Whether you're a parent wrangling kids, a student burning the midnight oil, or a professional navigating the demands of the workweek, I've crafted this nutrition guide with your hectic lifestyle in mind. This guide is not about quick fixes, rigid meal plans, or the latest diet craze. Instead, it's a holistic exploration of foundational nutrition principles. We'll cut through the noise, offering clarity on the essentials of nutrition, and empower you with knowledge to **make choices that are practical, health-conscious, and aligned with your unique lifestyle.**

FOUNDATIONS OF NUTRITION

Important Disclosure:
Before delving into the wealth of information provided in this nutrition guide, it's crucial to understand its scope and limitations. **This guide does not provide medical advice.** While the content presented here is based on sound nutritional principles and evidence-based research, it is not intended to replace professional medical advice, diagnosis, or treatment. Instead, the information provided in this guide lays the foundational knowledge that every individual would benefit to know about nutrition. By equipping individuals with essential nutritional principles, we strive to promote informed decision-making and lifelong health habits.

Nutrition is a highly individualized aspect of health, and what works for one person may not necessarily be suitable for another. Ultimately, your health is your responsibility. It's essential to take ownership of your health journey and make decisions that align with your unique needs and circumstances. Seek personalized advice from a qualified healthcare professional or registered dietitian who can provide tailored recommendations based on your individual health status, goals, and preferences. By acknowledging and understanding these disclosures, you can approach the information in this guide with clarity and confidence, empowering yourself to make informed choices that support your health and well-being. Let's embark on this journey to better nutrition together, armed with knowledge and a commitment to lifelong health.

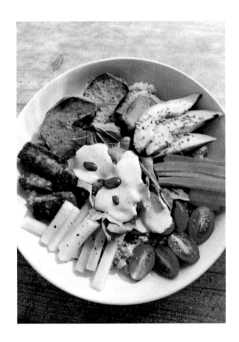

With all that said... I am excited to share with you the foundational principles of nutrition that will equip you with the tools to cultivate a nutritious, holistic lifestyle. I believe in empowering you with the knowledge and tools needed to make informed choices that align with your goals and preferences.

FOUNDATIONS OF NUTRITION

What To Expect:

1. **Foundations of Nutrition:** Let's dive into the basics – understanding macronutrients, decoding MyPlate recommendations, and mastering the art of reading nutrition labels. These are the building blocks that will empower you to make informed choices about what goes on your plate.

2. **Portion Sizes**: Discover the nuanced world of portion sizes. We'll explore how they vary based on your unique goals. This isn't about rigid meal plans; it's about understanding the flexibility and adaptability of your nutrition choices. Tailor your nutrition to meet your individual objectives, whether it's weight management, muscle building, or overall well-being.

3. **Meal Times**: Learning about what to eat and when to eat can significantly impact your energy levels, physical performance, and the quality of your sleep. By syncing your meals with your lifestyle, we'll optimize your nutrition for enhanced vitality. Discover how strategic timing can enhance your energy levels, support recovery, and optimize overall performance.

4. **Extra Goods**: Handouts created by me to make your life easier. Access practical tools designed to make your nutrition journey seamless.
   This includes:
   - A blank grocery shopping list to ensure your pantry is stocked with a diverse range of nutrient-dense foods.
   - A meal planning sheet to help you plan your week and create a roadmap for balanced, enjoyable meals.
   - Examples of high-protein snacks to keep you fueled and satisfied throughout your day.
   - Gain valuable tips on making mindful choices when dining out at restaurants.
   - Combining all of these tools together into a practical, realistic example that is flexible enough to fit your lifestyle.

This guide is not about handing you a one-size-fits-all meal plan. Instead, it's a holistic journey toward understanding and implementing the principles of nutrition that resonates with your lifestyle. It is your go-to companion for making nutrition work for you and not against you. By the end of this guide, my goal is for you to possess the knowledge and confidence to curate a nutritious way of life that aligns with your individual needs and goals.

Together, we will simplify the journey to a healthier you in the midst of life's beautiful chaos. Get ready to unlock the foundations of nutrition and pave the way towards a healthier, more vibrant you!

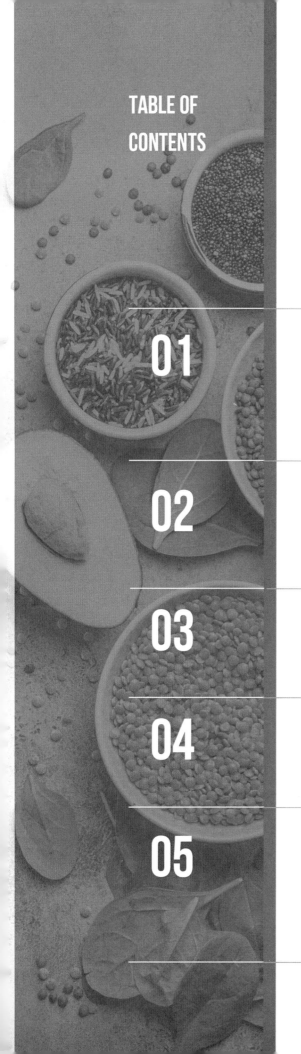

TABLE OF CONTENTS

FOUNDATIONS OF NUTRITION

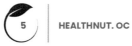

FOUNDATIONS OF NUTRITION

Understanding Macronutrients: Building Blocks for Your Body

In the world of nutrition, macronutrients – carbohydrates, protein, and fat – play pivotal roles in fueling our bodies and supporting daily functions. Let's break down the basics:

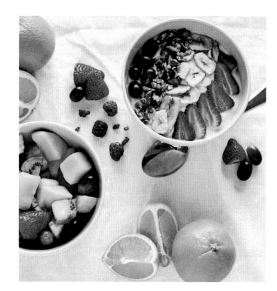

I. Carbohydrates:
The Brain's Best Friend

Carbohydrates (carbs) play a crucial role in our overall well-being and have often been unfairly labeled as the enemy. Carbs are not the adversary. Carbs are instrumental in the body's energy metabolism and provide several essential benefits for overall health and performance. Here's an overview of their role and benefits.

The role of carbohydrates include:

1. **Primary Energy Source:** Carbohydrates serve as the body and brain's primary and most efficient source of energy. Carbs power everything from basic bodily functions to high-intensity workouts. They are the unsung heroes that keep us going throughout the day. They are broken down into glucose, which is readily used by cells for fuel, particularly for the brain and muscles during exercise.
2. **Supporting Nutrient Digestion and Utilization:** Carbs aid in the digestion of other essential nutrients, such as protein, by providing a source of energy for the body's metabolic processes. They also stimulate the release of digestive enzymes that break down proteins into amino acids, facilitating their absorption in the small intestine.
3. **Glycogen Storage:** Excess glucose is converted into glycogen and stored in the liver and muscles. Glycogen serves as a reserve energy source, especially during periods of fasting or prolonged physical activity.
4. **Metabolic Regulation:** Carbs play a role in regulating metabolism, insulin secretion, and blood sugar levels. Consuming carbohydrates with fiber slows down digestion and absorption, promoting stable blood sugar levels and reducing the risk of insulin spikes and crashes.

FOUNDATIONS OF NUTRITION

The benefits of carbohydrates include:

1. **Energy Boost**: Consuming simple carbohydrates, like pretzels and fruit, before exercise provides a readily available source of energy, enhancing performance and delaying fatigue.
2. **Muscle Preservation**: Carbs spare protein from being used as an energy source, preserving muscle tissue and promoting muscle repair and growth.
3. **Enhanced Recovery**: Consuming carbohydrates post-exercise replenishes glycogen stores and facilitates muscle recovery by promoting protein synthesis and reducing muscle breakdown.
4. **Improved Mood and Cognitive Function**: Carbohydrates can positively influence mood and cognitive function by providing glucose to the brain, enhancing concentration, and promoting feelings of well-being.
5. **Digestive Health**: Carbohydrates from whole grains, fruits, and vegetables provide dietary fiber, which supports digestive health, prevents constipation, and reduces the risk of chronic diseases such as heart disease and diabetes.
6. **Satiety**: High-fiber carbohydrates promote feelings of fullness and satiety, helping to control appetite and prevent overeating.
7. **Nutrient Density**: Many carbohydrate-rich foods are also rich in essential vitamins, minerals, and phytonutrients, contributing to overall nutrient intake and health.

One key type of carbohydrate to focus on is fiber. According to the USDA, approximately 95% of Americans do not meet the recommended daily fiber intake, consuming only 10-15 grams instead of the suggested 25 grams for women and 38 grams for men. This shortfall can lead to a range of health issues, such as digestive problems and increased risks of heart disease and type 2 diabetes. Notably, around 74% of Americans experience digestive health problems, which are often linked to inadequate fiber consumption.

So, What is Fiber?

Fiber is a type of carbohydrate that your body cannot fully digest. Unlike sugars and starches that are broken down into glucose, fiber passes through your body relatively intact. There are two primary types of fiber:

1. **Soluble Fiber**: Dissolves in water and forms a gel-like substance in the gut. It helps lower cholesterol and blood sugar levels. Examples include oats, beans, apples, and citrus fruits.
2. **Insoluble Fiber**: Does not dissolve in water and adds bulk to the stool, aiding in the movement of material through the digestive system. It helps with constipation. Examples include whole grains, nuts, and vegetables like cauliflower, green beans, and potatoes.

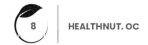

UNDERSTANDING MACRONUTRIENTS

Both types of fiber are essential as they play vital roles in the body, including:

- **Digestive Health**: Insoluble fiber helps with regularity, preventing constipation, while soluble fiber can alleviate diarrhea by firming up stool. Both fibers help balance digestion.
- **Heart Health**: Soluble fiber can help lower cholesterol levels by binding with bile acids (which contain cholesterol) in the intestine. Insoluble fiber aids in maintaining a healthy gut, which indirectly supports cardiovascular function.
- **Blood Sugar Control**: Soluble fiber slows the absorption of sugar which stabilizes blood sugar levels, a critical benefit for everyone, but especially for people with insulin resistance or diabetes.
- **Satiety and Weight Management**: Both types of fiber help increase feelings of fullness, which can aid in weight control by preventing overeating.

Soluble Fiber

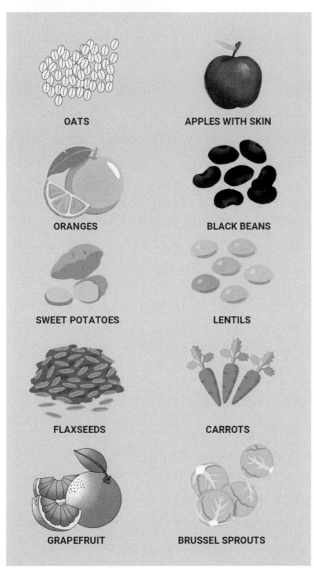

OATS   APPLES WITH SKIN

ORANGES   BLACK BEANS

SWEET POTATOES   LENTILS

FLAXSEEDS   CARROTS

GRAPEFRUIT   BRUSSEL SPROUTS

Insoluble Fiber

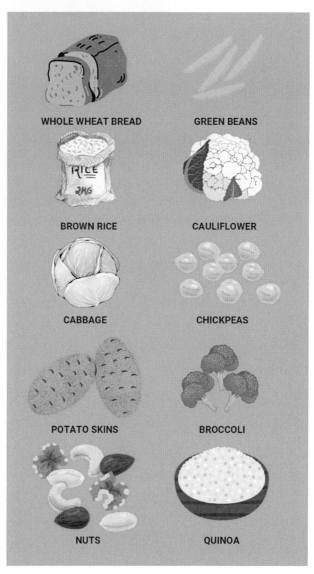

WHOLE WHEAT BREAD   GREEN BEANS

BROWN RICE   CAULIFLOWER

CABBAGE   CHICKPEAS

POTATO SKINS   BROCCOLI

NUTS   QUINOA

FOUNDATIONS OF NUTRITION

A balance of both insoluble and soluble fiber is applicable to nearly everyone. According to the Dietary Guidelines for Americans, the recommended daily intake for fiber is shown in the table below:

Recommended Daily Intake of Fiber	Ages 19 - 50	Ages 51+
Men	31 - 34 grams	28 grams
Women	25 - 28 grams	22 grams

However, specific amounts may vary depending on individual health goals and conditions. Consult a healthcare professional before making major dietary changes, especially if you have any specific medical conditions or sensitivities including:

- People with Digestive Sensitivities or Irritable Bowel Syndrome (IBS): Adjust fiber intake carefully, especially with insoluble fiber, which can aggravate symptoms. Soluble fiber from sources like oats and chia seeds is often better tolerated.
- People with Heart Disease or High Cholesterol: Soluble fiber can help reduce LDL (bad) cholesterol levels.
- People Managing Blood Sugar: Soluble fiber is helpful in slowing down the absorption of sugar, making it beneficial for people with prediabetes or diabetes.
- People Managing Weight: High-fiber foods increase satiety, making them beneficial for weight control.

*Important Note: It's crucial to slowly and gradually introduce more fiber into your diet to prevent side effects like gas, bloating, and diarrhea. Aim to increase fiber intake by about 5 grams every few days, and drink plenty of water to help the fiber move smoothly through your digestive system.

Tips to Increase Fiber Intake:
- **Choose Whole Grains:** Swap refined grains (white bread, jasmine rice, flour tortilla) for whole grains (whole wheat bread, brown rice, quinoa, corn tortilla).
- **Eat More Fruits and Vegetables:** Aim for a variety of fruits and vegetables, including those with edible skins, such as apples and potatoes.
- **Incorporate Beans and Legumes:** Add lentils, chickpeas, black beans, and other legumes into soups, salads, and main dishes.

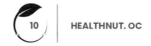

UNDERSTANDING MACRONUTRIENTS

- **Snack on Nuts and Seeds:** Choose high-fiber snacks like almonds, chia seeds, and flaxseeds.
- **Add Fiber-Rich Foods to Breakfast:** Include oats, whole-grain cereals, berries in your morning routine.

Fiber is an essential part of any diet, offering numerous health benefits beyond just digestive health. Prioritize fiber in your meals, and remember to increase it gradually to avoid discomfort. Fiber is just one component of a balanced diet, but its benefits extend far beyond digestion. While it's important to gradually increase your fiber intake for comfort, it's equally crucial to understand how different types of carbohydrates play a role in your overall nutrition.

As noted in Figure 1 on page 12, not all carbs are created equal. Consider the refined carbohydrate in a pastry – a delightful treat that provides a different purpose compared to whole-grain bread. Rather than pitting them against each other, recognize their unique roles. Pastries, rich in fat due to buttery goodness, may bring happiness, while whole-grain bread, packed with fiber, satisfies and supports digestion (which can also be delicious and bring us happiness).

The key lies in balance and understanding that each type of carbohydrate serves a purpose. Make room for both in your life, embracing the joy of pastries and the nourishment of whole-grain bread. It's not about one being better; it's about celebrating the diversity of carbs and their contributions to our daily vitality.

So, let's debunk the myth of carbs as the enemy and welcome them as essential partners in our journey to a balanced and vibrant lifestyle!

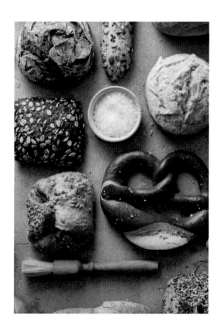 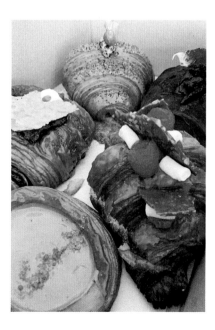 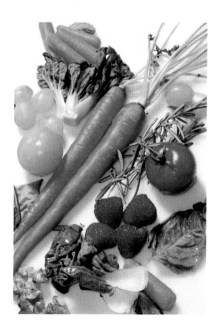

FIGURE I

Types of Carbohydrates

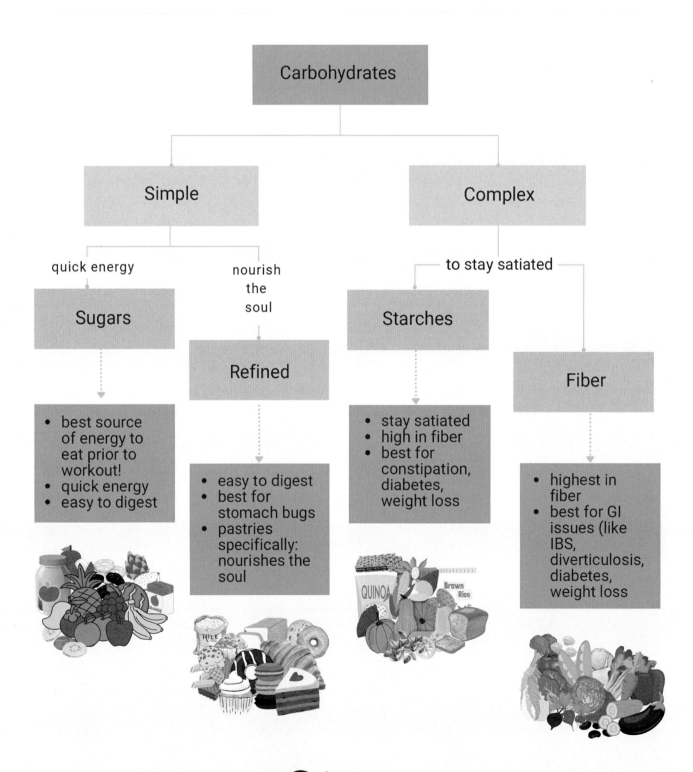

Carbohydrates

Simple

Complex

quick energy

nourish
the
soul

to stay satiated

Sugars

- best source of energy to eat prior to workout!
- quick energy
- easy to digest

Refined

- easy to digest
- best for stomach bugs
- pastries specifically: nourishes the soul

Starches

- stay satiated
- high in fiber
- best for constipation, diabetes, weight loss

Fiber

- highest in fiber
- best for GI issues (like IBS, diverticulosis, diabetes, weight loss

UNDERSTANDING MACRONUTRIENTS

II. Protein: The Power of Protein

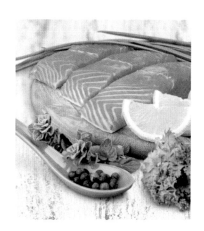

Protein – it's more than just a buzzword in the world of nutrition. You've likely heard of its importance, but let's dive deeper into why it's the cornerstone of a balanced diet and how we can leverage its benefits to fuel our busy lives.

The role of protein includes:

1. **Tissue Building and Repair**: Protein is essential for the growth, maintenance, and repair of tissues throughout the body, including muscles, organs, skin, hair, and nails. It provides the structural framework for cells and tissues, contributing to their strength, integrity, and function.
2. **Enzymes and Hormones**: Protein acts as catalysts for biochemical reactions in the body, serving as enzymes that facilitate various metabolic processes. Additionally, proteins function as hormones, regulating physiological functions such as growth, metabolism, and reproduction.
3. **Immune Function**: Many components of the immune system, including antibodies, cytokines, and immune cells, are made up of proteins. Protein plays a vital role in defending the body against pathogens, infections, and foreign invaders, contributing to overall immune function and resilience.
4. **Transport and Storage**: Certain proteins, such as hemoglobin and albumin, serve as carriers for transporting molecules like oxygen, nutrients, and hormones throughout the body. Proteins also play a role in storing essential nutrients and molecules for future use.
5. **Fluid Balance**: Proteins help maintain fluid balance within cells and tissues by regulating osmotic pressure and fluid distribution. For example, albumin, a protein in blood plasma, helps prevent fluid leakage from blood vessels and maintains blood volume and pressure.
6. **pH Balance**: Proteins act as buffers, helping to maintain the body's pH balance by absorbing or releasing hydrogen ions to stabilize the internal environment and support optimal physiological function.
7. **Muscle Function**: Protein is crucial for muscle contraction, strength, and repair. It provides the amino acids necessary for muscle protein synthesis, which is essential for muscle growth, maintenance, and recovery after exercise or injury.
8. **Energy Source**: While carbohydrates and fats are the body's primary sources of energy, protein can be metabolized for energy when carbohydrate and fat stores are depleted. However, protein is primarily used for structural and functional purposes rather than energy production.

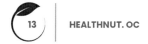

FOUNDATIONS OF NUTRITION

The benefits of proteins include:

1. **Muscle Building and Repair**: Protein provides the essential amino acids our bodies need to repair and build muscle tissue. Whether you're hitting the gym or simply going about your day, protein supports muscle recovery and growth.
2. **Satiety and Hunger Control**: Ever notice how a protein-rich meal leaves you feeling fuller for longer? That's because protein helps regulate appetite suppressant hormones, keeping hunger at bay and reducing the likelihood of mindless snacking.
3. **Blood Sugar Management**: Pairing protein with carbohydrates can help stabilize blood sugar levels, preventing the dreaded energy crash that often follows carb-heavy meals or snacks. This is especially crucial for sustained energy throughout the day.
4. **Metabolic Boost**: Protein has a higher thermic effect compared to carbohydrates and fats, meaning your body burns more calories digesting and metabolizing it. Incorporating protein into your meals can help rev up your metabolism.

Protein is a vital macronutrient with diverse functions essential for overall health, growth, and vitality. With the benefits of protein in mind, let's harness the power of protein to support our active lifestyles, manage hunger, and fuel our bodies for success. When it comes to mid-day snacking, pairing protein with another macronutrient (like carbs or healthy fats) creates a winning combination that leads to sustained energy, satiety satisfaction, and nutritional balance. With a little creativity and intentionality, we can elevate our snacking game and reap the rewards of a protein-rich diet. Some smart snacking options include Greek yogurt with berries, hard-boiled eggs with pretzels, and hummus with vegetables. Head to page 51 in the Appendix for more high-protein snack ideas!

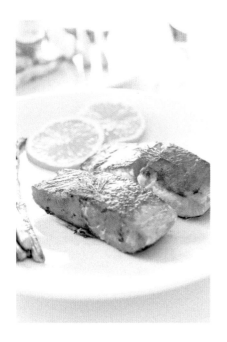 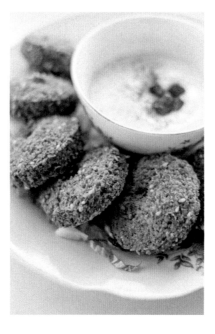 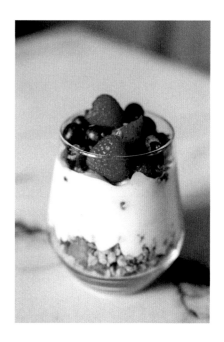

UNDERSTANDING MACRONUTRIENTS

III. Fat: Not All Fats Are Created Equal

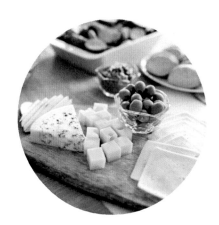

Despite its reputation, fat is crucial for optimal health, serving as a concentrated source of energy and aiding in the absorption of fat-soluble vitamins (vitamins A, D, E, and K). Not all fats are created equal, and understanding the difference can empower you to make healthier choices for your body. Let's delve into the world of fats and uncover their impact on your health.

To start, here's an overview of the role of fats:

1. **Energy Storage and Utilization**: Fats are the body's most concentrated source of energy, providing more than twice the energy per gram compared to carbohydrates and proteins. They serve as a stored energy reserve, providing fuel during periods of fasting or prolonged exercise.

2. **Cell Structure and Function**: Fats are integral components of cell membranes, contributing to their structure, flexibility, and function. Phospholipids, a type of fat that surrounds cells and helps regulate the passage of molecules in and out of cells.

3. **Hormone Production**: Fats are precursors to various hormones and signaling molecules, including steroid hormones such as testosterone, estrogen, and cortisol. These hormones play essential roles in regulating metabolism, growth, reproduction, and stress response.

4. **Absorption of Fat-Soluble Vitamins**: Fats facilitate the absorption of fat-soluble vitamins and other fat-soluble nutrients across the intestinal lining of the digestive tract and into the bloodstream for use by the body.

5. **Insulation and Temperature Regulation**: Adipose tissue, composed primarily of fat cells, acts as insulation, helping to maintain body temperature and protect internal organs from cold temperatures. Fats provide thermal insulation and help regulate heat exchange between the body and the environment.

6. **Organ Protection**: Fats provide cushioning and protection for vital organs, such as the heart, kidneys, and liver. Adipose tissue surrounding these organs helps absorb shock and minimize damage from external impacts.

7. **Brain Health**: Certain fats, particularly omega-3 fatty acids, are essential for brain development, cognitive function, and neurological health. They play a role in maintaining the structure and function of brain cell membranes and supporting neurotransmitter signaling.

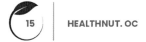

FOUNDATIONS OF NUTRITION

The benefits of fats include:

1. **Satiety and Appetite Regulation:** Fats contribute to feelings of fullness and satiety, helping to regulate appetite and reduce overeating. Including healthy fats in meals can promote greater satisfaction and longer-lasting energy levels.
2. **Heart Health**: Certain types of fats, such as monounsaturated and polyunsaturated fats found in nuts, seeds, avocados, and fatty fish, have been associated with improved heart health and reduced risk of cardiovascular disease when consumed in moderation.
3. **Skin and Hair Health**: Fats contribute to healthy skin and hair by providing essential fatty acids that support skin barrier function, moisture retention, and hair strength and shine.
4. **Mood Regulation**: Omega-3 fatty acids, in particular, have been linked to improved mood, reduced inflammation, and lower risk of depression and anxiety.
5. **Long-Term Energy**: Fats provide a sustained source of energy, especially during low-intensity activities or prolonged periods of exercise, making them valuable for endurance athletes and individuals engaged in long-duration activities.

There are also different types of fats. It's true — some fats can wreak havoc on your health, while others can help reduce inflammation and support overall well-being. Fats can be separated into two main categories: (1) saturated fats and (2) unsaturated fats. See Figure 2 on page 19 for a flowsheet visualizing the different types of fats.

1. **Saturated Fats** are solid at room temperature. Imagine what they do in your bloodstream once consumed. High consumption of saturated fats has been linked to an increased risk of heart disease, clogged arteries, and diabetes. These fats lurk in processed foods, fried goodies, and many packaged snacks, so it's essential to read labels and make informed choices.
2. **Unsaturated Fats** can be split into three subcategories, some more nutritious than others. These include trans fat, polyunsaturated fatty acids, and monounsaturated fatty acids.
   - **Trans Fat**, like saturated fat, should be consumed in moderation. Trans fats are a type of unsaturated fat that have been chemically altered through a process called hydrogenation, which makes them more solid and extends the shelf life of processed foods. These fats are commonly found in partially hydrogenated oils used in many fried foods, baked goods, and packaged snacks such as margarine, cookies, and crackers. Trans fats are harmful to health because they increase levels of LDL (bad) cholesterol while decreasing levels of HDL (good) cholesterol, leading to an elevated risk of heart disease, stroke, and type 2 diabetes. Reducing intake of trans fats is crucial for maintaining cardiovascular health and overall well-being.

UNDERSTANDING MACRONUTRIENTS

But fear not – the remaining types of unsaturated fats offer a host of benefits for your body and can be found in foods like avocados, nuts, seeds, and olive oil. These include polyunsaturated fatty acids (PUFAs) and monounsaturated fatty acids (MUFAs) which are considered healthy fats that offer various benefits for heart health and overall well-being. They can help lower bad cholesterol levels (LDL), reduce inflammation, and support heart health.

*Pro tip: Increase more unsaturated fats to support heart health, reduce inflammation, and promote overall well-being. You will then naturally decrease the amount of saturated fat and trans fat consumed.

- **Polyunsaturated Fatty Acids (PUFAs)** are essential fats that the body cannot produce on its own and must be obtained from the diet. They are known for their role in reducing LDL cholesterol levels and lowering the risk of cardiovascular disease. Examples of PUFAs include omega-3 and omega-6 fatty acids. Omega-3 fatty acids are renowned for their anti-inflammatory properties, which can help combat conditions like arthritis and promote brain health. They can be found in food sources like salmon, walnuts, and flaxseeds. Omega-6 fatty acids, found in vegetable oils and nuts, also play essential roles in the body but need to be balanced with omega-3s for optimal health.

The recommended ratio between omega-6 and omega-3 fatty acids is typically cited as 4:1 or less for optimal health. This ratio is important because both omega-6 and omega-3 fatty acids are essential for various physiological functions in the body, but they compete for the same enzymes in the metabolic pathway. A balanced ratio helps maintain proper immune function, reduce inflammation, support cardiovascular health, and promote overall well-being.

Excessive intake of omega-6 fatty acids, commonly found in processed foods and vegetable oils, can lead to chronic inflammation, which is linked to various diseases such as heart disease, diabetes, and arthritis. By aiming for a ratio of 4:1 or lower, individuals can help ensure a balanced intake of these essential fatty acids and mitigate the risk of inflammation-related health issues.

- **Monounsaturated Fatty Acids (MUFAs)** are known for their ability to improve blood cholesterol levels by raising HDL cholesterol (the "good" cholesterol) while lowering LDL cholesterol. MUFAs also offer anti-inflammatory properties and have been associated with reduced risk of heart disease, stroke, and diabetes. Including MUFAs in the diet may also help with weight management and promote feelings of fullness and satisfaction after meals. MUFAs are another type of healthy fat found in foods like olive oil, avocados, nuts, and seeds.

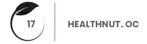

FOUNDATIONS OF NUTRITION

While unsaturated fats boast an impressive resume of health benefits, it's essential to practice moderation. Fat is more calorie-dense than other macronutrients. At nine calories per gram, they're the most energy-dense macronutrient. Therefore, while incorporating healthy fats into your diet is important, it's equally crucial to be mindful of portion sizes (more information in the next section). A little goes a long way - which is beneficial to know based on your nutrition goals.

The next time you hear the word "fat," think beyond the stereotypes. Embrace the power of healthy fats to fuel your body, protect your heart, and support overall wellness. With knowledge as your guide, you can make informed choices that nourish your body and enrich your life.

Combining all macronutrients into a balanced diet can indeed seem confusing and complicated, especially when some foods fall under multiple categories. See Figure 3 on page 20 to unravel the complexities of macronutrients. For example, beans are both a carbohydrate and a protein source. When using beans in your meals, it's essential to adjust the rest of your plate accordingly to maintain balance. Portion sizes will need to change based on how you are categorizing that food item - more information on this in the next section. While this might sound overwhelming, remember that the key to a healthy diet is nourishing your body and enjoying the positive effects of nutritious eating. Rather than getting bogged down by every detail, focus on making balanced choices and listening to your body's needs. If you're feeling better, more energized, and healthier, then you're already succeeding in your journey towards a balanced diet.

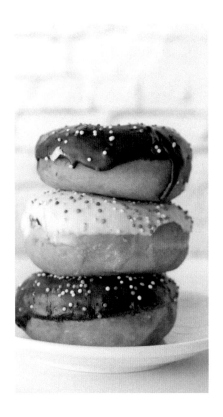
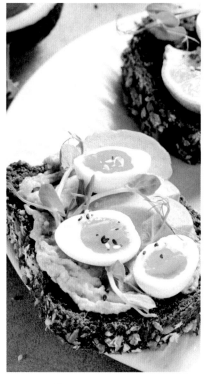
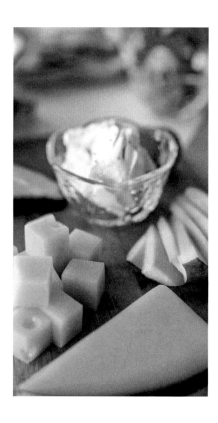

UNDERSTANDING MACRONUTRIENTS

FIGURE 2

Types of Fats

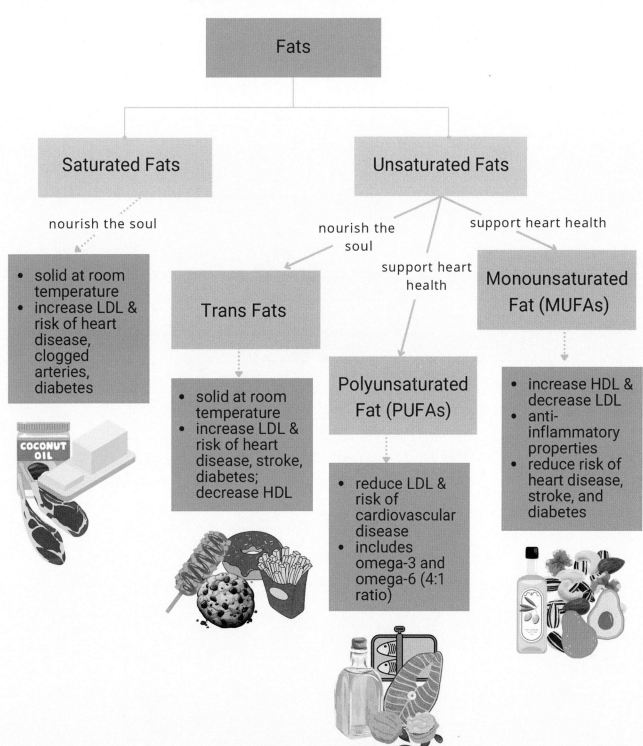

Fats

Saturated Fats

Unsaturated Fats

nourish the soul

- solid at room temperature
- increase LDL & risk of heart disease, clogged arteries, diabetes

nourish the soul

support heart health

support heart health

Trans Fats

- solid at room temperature
- increase LDL & risk of heart disease, stroke, diabetes; decrease HDL

Polyunsaturated Fat (PUFAs)

- reduce LDL & risk of cardiovascular disease
- includes omega-3 and omega-6 (4:1 ratio)

Monounsaturated Fat (MUFAs)

- increase HDL & decrease LDL
- anti-inflammatory properties
- reduce risk of heart disease, stroke, and diabetes

FOUNDATIONS OF NUTRITION

FIGURE 3

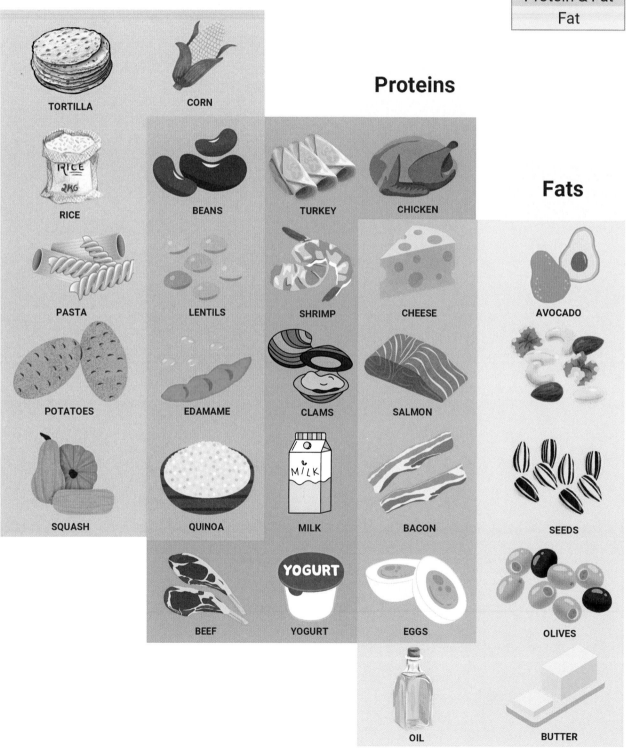

Carbs

Proteins

Fats

Legend
Carbs
Carbs & Protein
Protein
Protein & Fat
Fat

Carbs: TORTILLA, CORN, RICE, PASTA, POTATOES, SQUASH

Carbs & Protein: BEANS, LENTILS, EDAMAME, QUINOA, BEEF

Proteins: TURKEY, CHICKEN, SHRIMP, CLAMS, MILK, YOGURT

Protein & Fat: CHEESE, SALMON, BACON, EGGS

Fats: AVOCADO, SEEDS, OLIVES, OIL, BUTTER

PORTION SIZES - MASTERING MYPLATE

Portion Sizes
I. Mastering MyPlate: The Blueprint for Balanced Nutrition

Welcome to the MyPlate zone – your ticket to crafting meals that nourish and energize you from within. The MyPlate guidelines helps you include a variety of foods from different food groups, ensuring you get a wide range of vitamins, minerals, and other essential nutrients. But first, what is MyPlate?

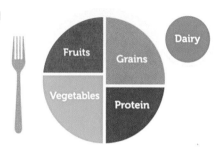

"MyPlate" is a visual representation of a healthy balanced diet developed by the United States Department of Agriculture (USDA). It replaced the MyPyramid food guidance system in 2011. MyPlate is designed to help individuals make healthier food choices and understand the proportions of different food groups to include in their meals. Here's a breakdown of the components of MyPlate:

1. **Plate Composition**: Picture your plate as a canvas, waiting to be adorned with a rainbow of nutrients. Each meal should include a balance of carbohydrates, protein, fruits, vegetables, and dairy products. This symphony of flavors and textures ensures you're getting a well-rounded mix of essential nutrients to fuel your body and mind. Try to make your plate look as colorful as possible to provide a wide range of vitamins, minerals, antioxidants, and phytochemicals.

2. **Fruit**: ¼ of the plate is dedicated to fruits. This includes fresh, frozen, canned, or dried fruits. MyPlate encourages variety and choosing fruits without added sugars whenever possible.

3. **Vegetables**: Another ¼ of the plate is allocated for vegetables. It emphasizes consuming a variety of colorful vegetables, including dark leafy greens, red and orange vegetables, legumes, and starchy vegetables like potatoes and corn.

4. **Grains**: The remaining ½ of the plate is divided between grains and protein foods. Grains take up slightly more space, emphasizing the importance of whole grains. This category includes foods like whole wheat bread, brown rice, oats, quinoa, and corn tortilla.

5. **Protein**: The protein section of MyPlate includes foods such as lean meats, poultry, seafood, eggs, nuts, seeds, and legumes like beans and peas. It's recommended to vary protein sources and choose lean or plant-based options more often.

6. **Dairy**: Outside of the plate, there's a smaller circle representing dairy, emphasizing the importance of consuming dairy or dairy alternatives for calcium and vitamin D. This includes milk, yogurt, cheese, and fortified plant-based alternatives.

See the next two pages to see what ingredients fall under each food group and ideas of nutrient-dense meals that follow MyPlate.

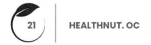

BUILD YOUR PLATE

Proteins

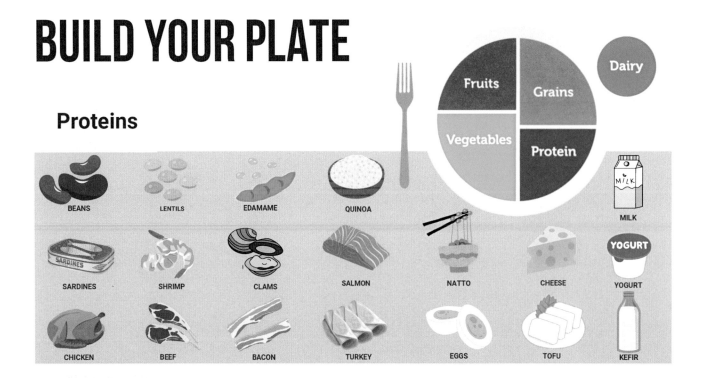

BEANS · LENTILS · EDAMAME · QUINOA · MILK
SARDINES · SHRIMP · CLAMS · SALMON · NATTO · CHEESE · YOGURT
CHICKEN · BEEF · BACON · TURKEY · EGGS · TOFU · KEFIR

Fruits · Grains · Dairy · Vegetables · Protein

Starches

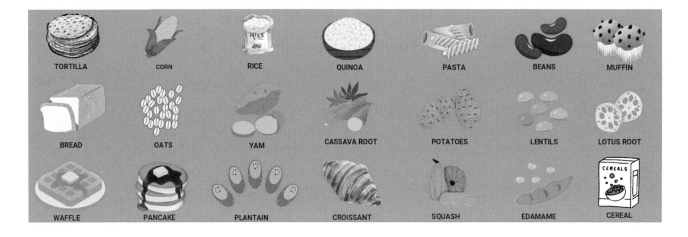

TORTILLA · CORN · RICE · QUINOA · PASTA · BEANS · MUFFIN
BREAD · OATS · YAM · CASSAVA ROOT · POTATOES · LENTILS · LOTUS ROOT
WAFFLE · PANCAKE · PLANTAIN · CROISSANT · SQUASH · EDAMAME · CEREAL

Fruits

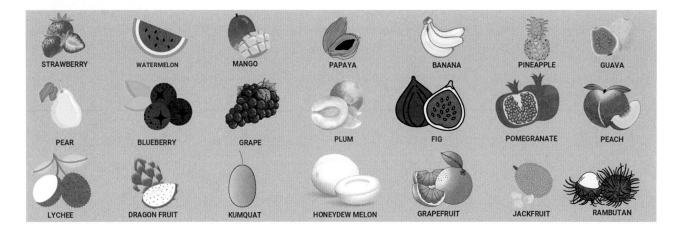

STRAWBERRY · WATERMELON · MANGO · PAPAYA · BANANA · PINEAPPLE · GUAVA
PEAR · BLUEBERRY · GRAPE · PLUM · FIG · POMEGRANATE · PEACH
LYCHEE · DRAGON FRUIT · KUMQUAT · HONEYDEW MELON · GRAPEFRUIT · JACKFRUIT · RAMBUTAN

BUILD YOUR PLATE

Vegetables

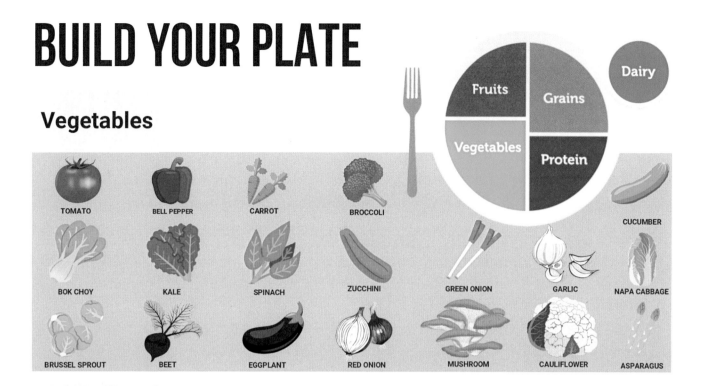

TOMATO BELL PEPPER CARROT BROCCOLI CUCUMBER
BOK CHOY KALE SPINACH ZUCCHINI GREEN ONION GARLIC NAPA CABBAGE
BRUSSEL SPROUT BEET EGGPLANT RED ONION MUSHROOM CAULIFLOWER ASPARAGUS

Fruits Grains Dairy
Vegetables Protein

Dairy

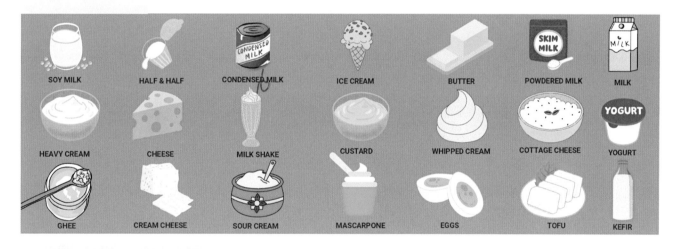

SOY MILK HALF & HALF CONDENSED MILK ICE CREAM BUTTER POWDERED MILK MILK
HEAVY CREAM CHEESE MILK SHAKE CUSTARD WHIPPED CREAM COTTAGE CHEESE YOGURT
GHEE CREAM CHEESE SOUR CREAM MASCARPONE EGGS TOFU KEFIR

Meal Examples

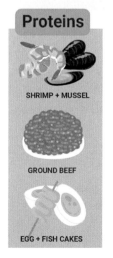 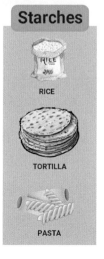 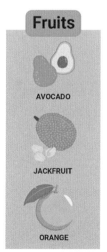 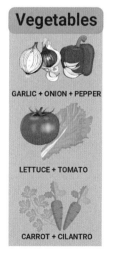 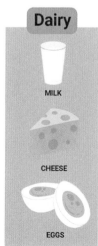 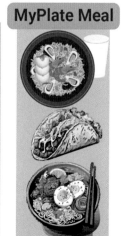

Proteins	Starches	Fruits	Vegetables	Dairy	MyPlate Meal
SHRIMP + MUSSEL	RICE	AVOCADO	GARLIC + ONION + PEPPER	MILK	
GROUND BEEF	TORTILLA	JACKFRUIT	LETTUCE + TOMATO	CHEESE	
EGG + FISH CAKES	PASTA	ORANGE	CARROT + CILANTRO	EGGS	

FOUNDATIONS OF NUTRITION

When using MyPlate as a guide for creating balanced meals, it's important to understand how to incorporate foods that count toward multiple macronutrient categories. Beans and cheese were discussed earlier in Figure 3 (page 20) as they fall under two food groups. Beans are considered proteins and carbs while cheeses are considered protein and fats. Here's one example on how to incorporate beans into your meal and adjust portion sizes accordingly:

If you use **beans** primarily as a **carbohydrate** source:
1. Fill 1/4 of your plate with beans as the carbohydrate.
2. Include a separate protein source, such as chicken, fish, tofu, or eggs, in the protein section of your plate.

If you choose to use **beans** primarily as your **protein** source:
1. Fill 1/4 of your plate with beans. The remaining 1/4 of the plate designated for protein can be omitted or reduced, as the beans fulfill this category.
2. Ensure the other 1/4 of your plate is filled with whole grains or other carbohydrate sources, like brown rice or quinoa.

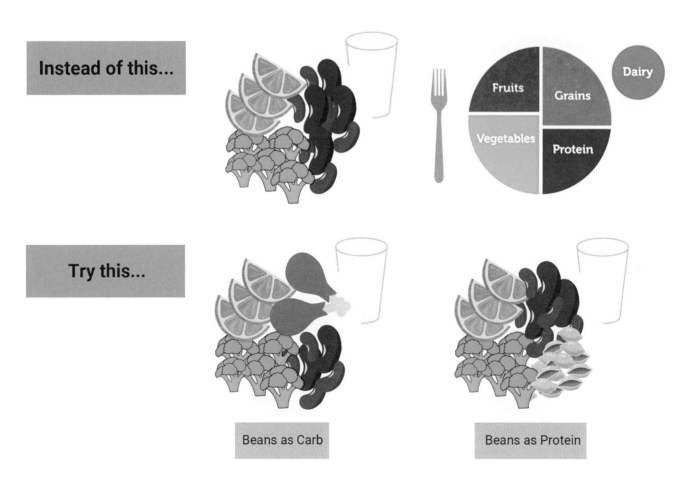

Instead of this...

Try this...

Beans as Carb

Beans as Protein

PORTION SIZES - MASTERING MYPLATE

Here's another example on how to incorporate cheese into your meal and adjust portion sizes accordingly:

If you use cheese primarily as a **protein** source:
1. Choose the variety of cheese that is higher in protein (like parmesan or cheddar).
2. Use larger portions of cheese and include a separate protein source, such as chicken, fish, tofu, or eggs, to help meet your protein needs.

Example: If adding cheese to a salad, you could use 2 oz of a high-protein cheese like parmesan or cheddar, while reducing the portion of chicken or legumes.

If you choose to use cheese primarily as your **fat** source:
1. Choose the variety of cheese that is richer in fat (like brie).
2. Use smaller portions of cheese to balance it with other protein sources like lean meat or plant-based proteins.

Example: If making a sandwich, you could use 1 oz of a higher-fat cheese like brie, while including turkey breast or tofu to provide the majority of the protein.

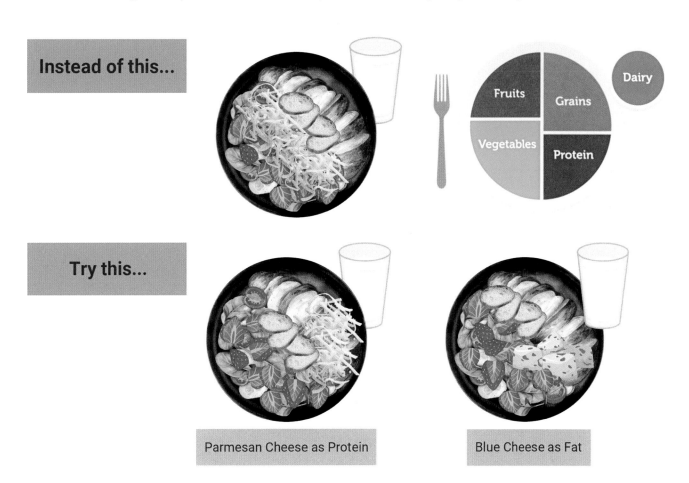

Instead of this...

Try this...

Parmesan Cheese as Protein

Blue Cheese as Fat

FOUNDATIONS OF NUTRITION

 MyPlate promotes healthy eating habits such as portion control, balancing calories, reducing sodium and added sugars, and drinking water instead of sugary beverages. It's a simple and practical tool to guide individuals toward a balanced and nutritious diet. But of course, things are never that simple. What makes it complicated is that food groups overlap. Take beans and legumes, for example, which straddle the line between protein and starch. When creating your plate, consider whether you're using them as your protein source or your starch source, and adjust portion sizes accordingly to ensure a balanced meal.

 The following table is a comparison of different types of beans and cheeses while strategically adjusting portion sizes based on nutrition goals:

Nutrition Goal	Serving Size	Food Example	Caloric Intake	Strategy
Gain Weight	1.5 - 2 cups	Kidney, Chickpeas	Higher Calories	Larger Portions, Higher-Calorie
	2 - 3 oz	Cheddar, Gouda		
Maintain Weight	1 cup	Black, Pinto	Moderate Calories	Moderate Portions, Balanced Intake
	1 - 2 oz	Mozzarella, Feta		
Become Leaner	1/2 - 3/4 cup	Lentils, Black	Lower Calories	Smaller Portions, Lower-Fat
	1 oz	Parmesan, Cottage		

PORTION SIZES - MASTERING MYPLATE

Portion sizes can be adjusted for health goals. Carbohydrate intake, in particular, may be adjusted based on weight goals. For those aiming for weight loss or maintenance, carbs should make up around a quarter of the plate. Conversely, for weight gain, carbs can comprise two-thirds to half of the plate. Listen to your body and adjust accordingly to support your goals. More information can be found in the section "Tailoring MyPlate: Adjusting Portion Sizes for Health Goals".

While it might seem complex to categorize and portion out food like beans and cheese, the key is to focus on the overall balance and variety of your meals. Don't get overwhelmed with the minute details. Instead, focus on balance, nourishment, and mindfulness. Aim for a balanced plate with a mix of different food group. Prioritize nourishing your body with wholesome, nutrient-dense foods. Pay attention to how your body feels and adjust portions based on your hunger, energy levels, and dietary needs.

As long as you are eating a variety of foods and noticing positive effects on your health and well-being, you are already on the right track. Enjoy your meals and focus on creating a sustainable, healthy eating pattern rather than getting tangled by every detail.

A well-balanced meal isn't just about checking off boxes — it's about reaping the rewards of vibrant health and vitality. From steady energy levels and improved mood to enhanced digestion and better weight management, the benefits are endless when you prioritize balance on your plate. Further details listed below:

- **Nutrient Intake**: Each food group provides different nutrients essential for overall health. By including all food groups, you ensure you're meeting your body's nutritional needs.
- **Sustained Energy**: A balanced meal provides a steady release of energy throughout the day, helping to prevent energy crashes and fatigue.
- **Weight Management**: Balancing portion sizes and food choices can aid in weight management by controlling calorie intake and promoting satiety.
- **Improved Digestion**: Including a variety of fiber-rich foods such as fruits, vegetables, and whole grains supports healthy digestion.
- **Better Mood and Mental Clarity**: Balanced meals can contribute to stable blood sugar levels, which in turn can help regulate mood and improve cognitive function.

With MyPlate as your guide, you have the power to create meals that nourish your body and soul. Keep it simple, embrace variety, and remember to savor the journey — because when it comes to nutrition, balance is the key to unlocking your fullest potential. By following these guidelines and finding a balance between enjoyment and health, you can create sustainable habits that support your overall well-being.

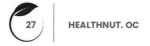

FOUNDATIONS OF NUTRITION

With all of this information, it is important to find balance without obsession. Nutrition is a journey, not a destination – and it's essential to find a balance that works for you. While it's tempting to dive into the world of meticulous calorie counting and macronutrient tracking, remember to leave room for flexibility and enjoyment. Given busy lifestyles, sometimes frozen meals, takeout, or ready-to-eat options are the most convenient way to prepare meals. Finding a balance in nutrition means recognizing that sometimes convenience is necessary, and that's okay. Focus on enhancing your meals with nutrient-dense foods as shown in the examples below. Remember that flexibility and enjoyment are key components of a sustainable and healthy lifestyle.

Nutrient-Dense Add-On Examples

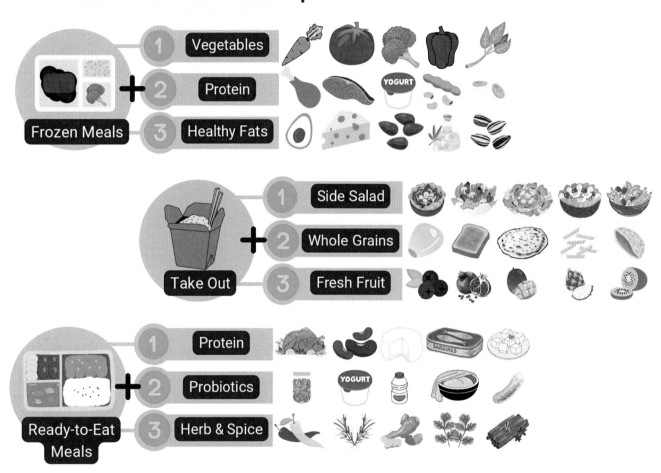

Alternatively, the hand method can serve as a handy tool for estimating portions on the fly, allowing you to enjoy your meals without the stress of constant calculation. More information on the hand method presented in the next section "Hand Method for Portion Sizes." Keep in mind that an occasional treat is not only okay but encouraged as part of a sustainable lifestyle. Cutting out favorite foods entirely can lead to cravings and binge eating. It's more effective to include them in moderation, without feeling guilty.

PORTION SIZES - HAND METHOD

Portion Sizes
II. Hand Method for Portion Sizes

While portion sizes may vary based on individual health goals and activity levels, a general guideline can help steer you in the right direction. The hand method is a simple and practical way to estimate portion sizes without the need for measuring tools or scales. It utilizes the size of your hand as a reference point for different food groups, making it easy to visualize and apply in various eating situations.

Here's how it works:

Proteins – Palm: Your palm size represents a serving of protein. This could include meats, poultry, fish, tofu, or beans. One portion of protein should be about the size of a palm and as thick as a deck of cards.

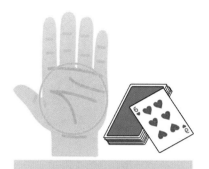

Proteins - 3 oz

Carbohydrates – Fist: Your closed fist represents a serving of carbohydrates. This includes foods like rice, pasta, bread, fruits, or cooked vegetables. One portion of raw fruits and cooked vegetables should be about the size of a clenched fist. A portion of starches should be about the size of half of a clenched first.

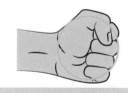

Carbohydrates - 1 cup

Raw Vegetables – Two Cupped Hands: Two cupped hands represent a serving of raw, leafy vegetables. This includes vegetables like spinach and lettuce.

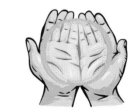

Raw Vegetables - 1 cup

Fats – Thumb: Your thumb size represents a serving of fats. This includes sources like oils, butter, or nuts.

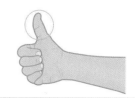

Fats - 1 tablespoon

General Guidelines - Hand Portions Per Meal		
	Protein	1-2 palms
	Vegetable	1-2 fists
	Carbohydrate	1-2 cupped handfuls
	Fat	1-2 thumbs

FOUNDATIONS OF NUTRITION

The advantages of the Hand Method includes simplicity, portability, adaptability, and visual cues. The hand method is easy to remember and doesn't require any special tools or equipment. Since it relies on the size of your hand, you can use this method anywhere, whether at home, work, or dining out. The hand method can be adjusted based on individual needs and preferences, making it suitable for various dietary preferences and health goals. It provides a visual cue for portion sizes, helping to prevent overeating and promote portion control.

By using the hand method to estimate portion sizes, individuals can develop a better understanding of balanced eating habits and make informed choices about their food intake without the need for strict calorie counting or measuring every meal.

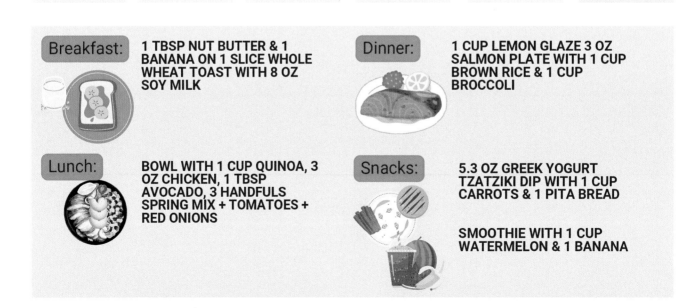

Food Group Example - 1,800 Calorie Plan

Proteins	Starches	Fruits	Vegetables	Fats	Nutrients
5 PALMS = 15 OZ	4 FISTS = 4 CUPS	3 FISTS = 3 CUPS	1 HANDFUL + 1.5 FISTS = 1 CUP RAW + 1.5 CUP COOKED VEGETABLES	3 THUMBS = 3 TBSP	1800 KCALS / 115 G PROTEIN / 200 G CARBS / 50 G FAT / 30 G FIBER

Breakfast: 1 TBSP NUT BUTTER & 1 BANANA ON 1 SLICE WHOLE WHEAT TOAST WITH 8 OZ SOY MILK

Dinner: 1 CUP LEMON GLAZE 3 OZ SALMON PLATE WITH 1 CUP BROWN RICE & 1 CUP BROCCOLI

Lunch: BOWL WITH 1 CUP QUINOA, 3 OZ CHICKEN, 1 TBSP AVOCADO, 3 HANDFULS SPRING MIX + TOMATOES + RED ONIONS

Snacks: 5.3 OZ GREEK YOGURT TZATZIKI DIP WITH 1 CUP CARROTS & 1 PITA BREAD

SMOOTHIE WITH 1 CUP WATERMELON & 1 BANANA

PORTION SIZES - TAILORING MYPLATE

Portion Sizes
III. Tailoring MyPlate: Adjusting Portion Sizes for Health Goals

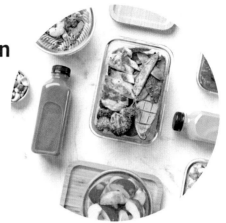

In line with the principles of MyPlate, portion sizes of food groups and macronutrients can be adjusted based on specific health goals, similar to the concept of an Athlete's Plate. The Athlete's Plate is tailored to meet the increased energy and nutrient needs of athletes and active individuals. Similarly, adjustments can be made to to macronutrient distribution within the framework of MyPlate to align with various health goals, such as weight loss, weight maintenance, muscle building, or performance optimization. The following explains how portion sizes may change based on different health objectives:

Weight Loss/Maintenance:
1. Carbohydrates: Carbs should constitute a smaller portion of the plate, around ¼ of the plate, to control calorie intake and promote fat loss or maintenance of a healthy weight.
2. Protein: Protein intake remains essential for preserving lean muscle mass during weight loss. Aim for a moderate portion of protein, roughly the size of your palm, to support satiety and muscle maintenance.
3. Fruits and Vegetables: Fill half of your plate with a variety of colorful fruits and vegetables to provide essential vitamins, minerals, and fiber while keeping calorie intake in check.
4. Dairy Products: Include a serving of dairy, such as a glass of milk or a serving of yogurt, for calcium and other nutrients essential for bone health.

Muscle Building/Performance Optimization:
1. Carbohydrates: Increase carb intake to fuel high-intensity workouts and replenish glycogen stores. Carbs should make up a larger portion of the plate, around 2/3 to ½ of your plate, to support energy needs.
2. Protein: Increase protein intake to support muscle repair and growth. Aim for a larger portion of protein, potentially exceeding the size of your palm, particularly after exercise sessions.
3. Fruits and Vegetables: Continue to fill half of your plate with fruits and vegetables to provide antioxidants and other micronutrients crucial for recovery and overall health.
4. Dairy Products: Include dairy sources for protein and calcium, which are important for muscle function and bone health.

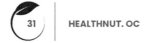

FOUNDATIONS OF NUTRITION

Weight Management Goals	Men	Female
Gain Weight (Increase Muscle)	+ 400 to 500 kcals/day	+ 300 to 400 kcals/day
Lose Weight (Decrease Fat)	- 300 to 500 kcals/day	- 200 to 300 kcals/day

Weight Gain

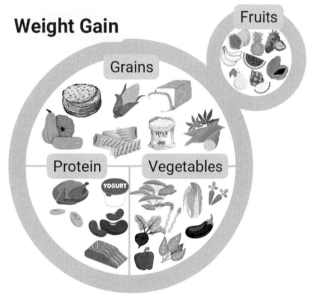

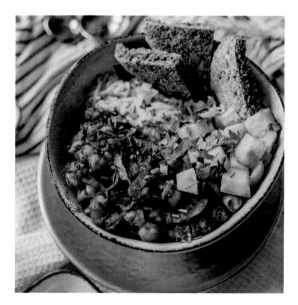

Weight Loss

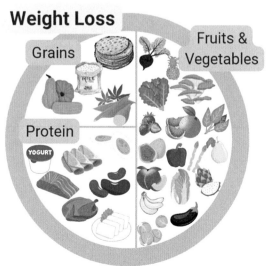

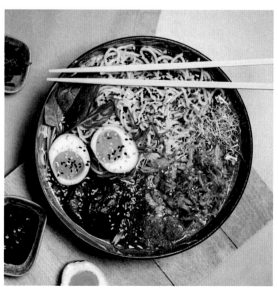

PORTION SIZES - TAILORING MYPLATE

The number of calories provided in the table above is an estimate and may vary depending on individual factors such as metabolism, activity level, and body composition. It's important to note that greater reductions in energy intake for weight loss may compromise energy levels and physical performance, while excessive increases for weight gain may lead to unwanted fat gain.

A reasonable weight loss goal is typically around 0.7% of body weight per week to ensure sustainable results without sacrificing muscle mass. For simultaneous muscle gain and fat loss, precise energy intake and nutrient timing are crucial, with adjustments often necessary in increments of 50 to 100 kcal per day until desired outcomes are achieved. Close monitoring and consultation with a healthcare professional or dietitian are recommended for optimal results.

Summary of Macronutrient Distribution	

Protein	**Not clearly defined, estimated to range from 1.5 - >2.0 g/kg**
	• Leucine, a branch-chained amino acid, is particularly important for initiating muscle protein synthesis, particularly when combined with resistance training.
	• Recommended amounts of Leucine for optimal muscle protein synthesis:
	    ○ Adult athletes: approximately 20-25 g/day
	    ○ Older athletes: approximately 30-40 g/day
	• Food sources rich in leucine include poultry, beef, pork, fish, dairy products such as yogurt and cheese, soy products like tofu, legumes such as beans and lentils, and nuts and seeds like almonds and pumpkin seeds

Carbohydrate	Approximately 3-12 g/kg
Fat	Approximately 1 g/kg or approximately 25-30% of total kcals

FOUNDATIONS OF NUTRITION

With all weight management goals, it is important to stay mindful of the foundations of nutrition, consistently referring back to MyPlate guidelines and understanding the nutrient composition of macronutrients. Ensuring a balanced intake of protein, carbohydrates, and fats will help support these goals while promoting overall health and performance.

Quick Note of Why Excess Protein Isn't Better:
While protein is crucial for muscle repair, recovery, and preserving lean body mass, more protein isn't necessarily better. The body can only use a certain amount of protein for muscle repair and other functions. When protein intake exceeds the body's needs:

1. **Storage as Fat:** Any excess protein not used for tissue repair or other bodily functions gets converted into glucose through a process called gluconeogenesis. If this glucose isn't used for energy, it is eventually stored as fat.
2. **Excretion of Nitrogen:** The body breaks down protein into amino acids, which contain nitrogen. Excess nitrogen gets processed by the liver and excreted by the kidneys as urea. This places additional strain on the kidneys and increases water loss, potentially leading to dehydration if fluid intake is not sufficient.

General Guidelines:
- **Hydration:** Regardless of health goals, staying hydrated is crucial for overall health and performance. Drink plenty of water throughout the day, and consider sports drinks or electrolyte beverages during intense workouts.
- **Balanced Approach:** While adjustments can be made to portion sizes, strive for balance and variety within each food group to ensure you're meeting all of your nutritional needs.
- **Individual Variation:** Portion sizes may vary based on individual factors such as age, gender, activity level, and metabolic rate. Experimentation and listening to your body's cues are key to finding the right balance for your unique needs.

It's crucial to emphasize that these dietary adjustments should be made during training periods, rather than during game seasons when peak performance is paramount. By adapting portion sizes within the MyPlate framework to align with specific health goals, individuals can optimize their nutrition to support their desired outcomes, whether it's weight management, muscle building, or performance enhancement.

NUTRIENT TIMING

Optimizing Your Nutrition:
A Lifestyle Aligned with Your Schedule

Creating a nutrition plan that synchronizes seamlessly with your lifestyle involves considering the timing of your meals in relation to exercise, sleep, and daily activities. Here's a guide to help you cultivate a personalized approach that caters to your unique schedule:

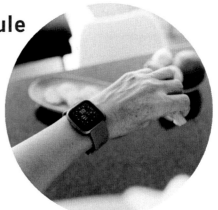

1. Prioritize Balanced Meals 3x/day:

- Eat breakfast! Eat within 1-2 hours of waking to keep your energy levels up. Cortisol is an essential hormone that affects the body's organs and tissues. It plays a role in stress, metabolism, and blood glucose levels to name a few. Cortisol levels naturally rise in the morning. If breakfast is skipped, cortisol level will not rise as it should, forcing you to start your day at lower energy levels.
- Don't skip dinner! Eating after 6pm does not automatically cause weight gain. This became a mainstream statement because it is recommended to not eat a full meal 2 hours before sleeping as late-night digestion will interrupt sleeping patterns - timing alone is not a direct cause of weight gain.
  - If you find yourself hungry before bedtime, a high-protein bedtime snack may be beneficial. Opt for options like Greek yogurt, cottage cheese, nuts, or edamame to satisfy hunger without overloading your digestive system.
- Instead of fixating on the clock, prioritize the content of your meals. Aim for a balanced meal that includes lean protein, fiber-rich carbohydrates, and healthy fats. This combination helps keep you satisfied, stabilizes blood sugar levels, and supports overall health. Refer back to the "Foundations of Nutrition" section for more detail and information.

2. Snack In-Between Meals:

- Stave off hunger and prevent overeating during mealtime by snacking strategically between meals. Strategic snacking includes combining protein with another macronutrient like whole-grain carbohydrates or healthy fats.
- Incorporating protein-rich snacks throughout the day can give your metabolism a gentle nudge, helping it run more efficiently and potentially aiding in weight management efforts.
- High-protein snacks provide a steady stream of energy, helping to keep blood sugar levels stable between meals. This translates to sustained focus, improved mood, and enhanced overall energy levels throughout the day.

FOUNDATIONS OF NUTRITION

- Wake up hungry or experience blood sugar fluctuations during the night? Grab a high-protein bedtime snack to provide sustained energy and help prevent midnight cravings without disrupting sleep.

3. Pre-Exercise Nutrition:
- Consume a balanced meal or snack 3-4 hours before a workout, providing a combination of carbohydrates, protein, and healthy fats for sustained energy.
- If exercising within 1-2 hours, opt for a smaller, easily digestible snack such as a banana, pickles, or pretzels.
  - Limit the amount of protein and fat 1-2 hours prior to exercise to prevent gastrointestinal distress. The recommended intake varies per individual; additionally, more research is required.
- If you are unable to eat breakfast before early morning exercise, consuming about 30 grams of easily digestible carbs 5 mins before exercise may improve performance.

How to use the following table:
1. Determine how many hours you are prior to your workout, then consume the corresponding amount of carbs from the table. For example, if a 130 lbs individual has 1 hour before exercise, aim to consume about 60 grams of carbs. The actual amount may vary depending on factors like individual metabolism, exercise intensity, and personal preferences.
2. Additionally, aim to choose easily digestible carbohydrates that won't cause gastrointestinal discomfort during exercise. Remember to hydrate adequately before, during, and after exercise. This helps to fuel your body adequately for optimal performance during your workout. Adjust portion sizes based on individual preferences and tolerances.

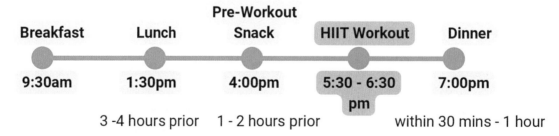

Example

Create a **pre-workout meal plan for Timmy, a 180 lb (82 kg) male who has an hour long high-intensity training workout planned at 5:30 pm.** We will consider the timing of his meals, aiming to ensure optimal fueling while avoiding gastrointestinal discomfort. His meals and snacks will be spaced out according to the timing of his workout.

NUTRIENT TIMING

Timing Before Exercise	Recommended Carbohydrate Intake (g/kg)	Example for a 130 lb / 59 kg Individual	Example of Carbohydrates with Portion Sizes
1 hour	1	59 g	17 mini pretzels + 1 carb energy gel
2 hours	2	118 g	4 fig cookie bars + 1 medium apple + 1 cup vanilla soy milk
3 hours	3	177 g	6 inch sandwich + 3 oz tortilla chips + ¼ cup salsa + 2 large oranges
4 hours	4	236 g	1 cup black beans and rice + 1 cup peas + ½ cup corn + 1 ½ cup chicken noodle soup + 1 cup apple juice + 2 cups strawberries + 6 oz plain yogurt

4. Post-Exercise Nutrition:
- Refuel with a combination of carbohydrates and 20-30 grams of protein within 30-60 mins after exercise to support muscle recovery.
- Examples include a protein smoothie, Greek yogurt with granola and berries, or a chicken wrap with veggies.

5. Adapt to Your Daily Routine:
- Align your main meals with your daily schedule. For those with irregular working hours, plan meals accordingly to maintain consistency.
- Carry healthy snacks, like nuts or fruit, to curb hunger and avoid making less nutritious choices when you're on the go.

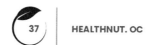

FOUNDATIONS OF NUTRITION

6. Mindful Eating for Better Digestion:
- Allow at least 20-30 minutes for each meal, focusing on mindful eating to aid digestion. While dining, sit down in a chair, eat without distractions, chew foods thoroughly, and enjoy your meal!
- Avoid large meals right before bedtime to prevent discomfort and disturbances in your sleep.

7. Prioritize Sleep:
- Aim for 7-9 hours of quality sleep each night, as insufficient sleep can disrupt hunger hormones and impact overall well-being.
- Avoid heavy or spicy meals close to bedtime to promote better sleep quality.

8. Hydration Throughout the Day:
- Stay hydrated by sipping water consistently throughout the day. Keep a water bottle with you at all times.
- Adjust your water intake based on factors like exercise intensity, climate, and individual needs.

9. Plan Ahead for Busy Days:
- Prepare and pack meals or snacks for busy days to ensure you have nutritious options readily available.
- Batch cooking or meal prepping on days with more time can streamline your nutrition on busier days.

10. Regular Check-ins and Adjustments:
- Periodically assess how your current eating schedule aligns with your lifestyle and adjust as needed.
- Consider consulting with a registered dietitian for personalized guidance based on your specific goals and preferences.

By integrating these practices into your daily routine, you can create a nutrition plan that complements your lifestyle, providing sustained energy, promoting optimal performance during exercise, and supporting restful sleep. Remember, individual needs vary, so embrace the flexibility to tailor these guidelines to your personal schedule and preferences. See the Appendix for extra practical handouts to help plan out your lifestyle and fueling schedule!

NUTRITION LABEL

Deciphering Nutrition Labels:
Your Guide to Informed Choices

Navigating the aisles of the grocery store can feel like a daunting task, especially when faced with rows of products competing for your attention. But fear not – armed with the knowledge of how to read nutrition labels, you can make confident, informed choices that support your health goals. Let's break down the key components of a nutrition label and empower you to make the best choices for your body.

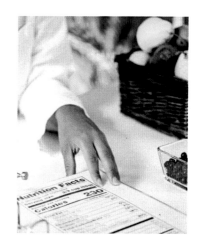

Nutrition labels – they're like mini roadmaps guiding you through the nutritional landscape of packaged foods. But without a bit of decoding, they can be overwhelming. Let's break it down step by step, so you can confidently navigate the aisles and make choices that align with your health goals:

1. **Serving sizes** listed on a nutrition label is not necessarily the recommended amount to eat in one sitting. Instead, it represents the standard portion size used for calculating nutritional information. Pay attention to this serving size, as all the nutrient values listed below correspond to this serving size.
2. **Calories** provide a snapshot of the energy content in one serving of the food. Understanding calorie counts is essential regardless of your nutrition goals. Whether you're aiming for weight loss, maintenance, or gain, being mindful of calorie content can help you make informed decisions about portion sizes and overall intake.
3. **Nutrients and % Daily Value** are found beneath the calorie count where you'll find a breakdown of various nutrients present in the food. This includes macronutrients like fat, protein, and carbohydrates, as well as micronutrients like vitamins and minerals. These values represent the amount of each nutrient in one serving of the food.

The % Daily Value (DV) indicates how much a serving of the food contributes to your daily recommended intake based on a 2,000-calorie diet. A handy rule of thumb: 5% or less of the % DV means the food is low in that nutrient, while 20% or more means it's high. For instance, if a food has 25% DV of sodium, it's considered high in sodium. Use this information to steer clear of excessive amounts of nutrients like saturated fat, sodium, and added sugars.

FOUNDATIONS OF NUTRITION

Keep in mind that your individual nutrient needs may vary based on factors such as age, sex, activity level, and health status. Consulting with a registered dietitian can provide personalized guidance.

Armed with this knowledge, you are now equipped to make informed decisions about the foods you consume. By being mindful of serving sizes, calories, nutrients, and %DV, you can take control of your nutritional intake and support your overall well-being. So, next time you're perusing the grocery aisles, let nutrition labels be your trusted guide to better eating habits.

Serving Information: servings in entire package & size of each serving

Nutrients:
Total Fat - total amount of saturated ('bad') fat and unsaturated ('good') fat in one serving.

Sugars - The amount of sugar naturally in product and how much is added.

Nutrients: Key nutrients in one serving of food

Nutrition Facts

Serving Size 10 oz.
Serving Per Container 5

Amount Per Serving

Calories 200   **Calories From Fat 200**

	% Daily value *
Total Fat 10g	35%
Saturated Fat 1.5g	11%
Trans Fat 0.0g	
Cholesterol 0 mg	1%
Sodium 210 mg	15%
Total Carbohydrate 15g	3%
Dietary Fiber 2g	3%
Sugars 3g	
Includes 2g Added Sugars	1%
Protein 30g	

Vitamin D 3mcg	10%
Calcium 260mg	20%
Iron 8mg	45%

*The % Daily Value (DV) tell you how much a nutrient in a serving of food contributes to a daily diet. 2,000 calories a day is used for general nutrition advice.

Calories: amount of energy from one serving

% Daily Value: The amount a nutrient contributes to a 2,000 calorie diet.

5% or less is **low** in that nutrient.

20% or more is **high** in that nutrient.

FREQUENTLY ASKED QUESTIONS

Frequently Asked Questions (FAQ)

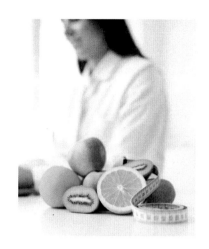

1. What is the best diet for weight loss?
There isn't a one-size-fits-all answer. The best diet for weight loss depends on individual preferences, health conditions, and lifestyle. However, generally, a balanced diet with plenty of fruits, vegetables, lean proteins, and whole grains is recommended. A couple diets I recommend are the Mediterranean diet and intermittent fasting. Keep reading down to question 4 and 5 for more information.

2. Are there any quick fixes for weight loss?
Quick fixes or fad diets often promise rapid weight loss but are not sustainable or healthy in the long term. Fad diets lead to slowed metabolism, yo-yo dieting, and increased risk of chronic diseases. It's important to focus on making gradual, sustainable changes to your eating habits in order to create a healthy lifestyle with lasting results.

3. Should I count calories?
Calorie counting can be a helpful tool for some people, especially those with specific weight goals, but it's not necessary for everyone. A more intuitive approach, such as focusing on portion control, eating nutrient-dense foods, and paying attention to hunger and fullness cues, can be equally effective. For many, building a balanced plate with protein, healthy fats, and fiber-rich carbs is a better long-term strategy than counting every calorie.

4. Do detox diets work?
Detox diets claim to rid the body of toxins and promote weight loss, but there's little scientific evidence to support their effectiveness. The weight loss observed from detox diets is often attributed to fluid loss and a decrease in caloric intake rather than sustainable fat loss. Once the detox period ends and normal eating resumes, the lost weight is likely to return, often accompanied by additional pounds due to rebound overeating or slowed metabolism. Detox diets rarely provide long-term solutions for weight management and may even promote unhealthy attitudes towards food and body image. The body has its own natural detoxification processes, primarily carried out by the liver and kidneys. Eating a balanced diet rich in fruits, vegetables, and whole foods supports these processes.

FOUNDATIONS OF NUTRITION

5. What is the Mediterranean diet and who would benefit from it?
The Mediterranean diet is a dietary pattern inspired by the traditional eating habits of people living in countries bordering the Mediterranean Sea. It typically includes abundant consumption of fruits, vegetables, whole grains, legumes, nuts, and olive oil, moderate intake of fish and poultry, and limited consumption of red meat and processed foods.

This diet is characterized by its anti-inflammatory properties, attributed to the high intake of antioxidants and omega-3 fatty acids found in its key components. Research suggests that adhering to the Mediterranean diet may reduce the risk of chronic diseases such as heart disease, diabetes, and certain cancers, while also promoting longevity and overall well-being. Individuals looking to improve their cardiovascular health, manage inflammation, and potentially increase their lifespan may benefit from adopting the Mediterranean diet.

6. What is intermittent fasting, and is it safe?
Intermittent fasting involves cycling between periods of eating and fasting. It can be safe for many people and may offer health benefits such as weight loss and improved metabolic health. However, it's important to approach intermittent fasting with caution, especially for individuals with certain medical conditions or eating disorders.

There are also different types of intermittent fasting. I recommend the 16:8 intermittent fasting method which involves fasting for 16 hours each day and eating all your meals within an 8-hour window. Typically, people choose to eat between noon and 8 PM. For optimal results, adopt a nutritious eating pattern during the 8-hour eating window rather than increasing the amounts of high-sugar, processed, and fried foods. During the 16-hour fasting period, only non-caloric beverages like water, tea, and black coffee are allowed. Focus on balanced meals that include plenty of fruits, vegetables, lean proteins, and whole grains to enhance the positive effects of the 16:8 intermittent fasting diet.

Fasting longer than 12 hours a day can lead to several negative consequences for both physical and mental health including weakness, dizziness, irritability, decreased energy levels, difficulty concentrating, and impaired cognitive function.

7. Is gluten-free diet beneficial for everyone?
A gluten-free diet is necessary for individuals with celiac disease or gluten sensitivity. For others, there's no evidence to suggest that eliminating gluten from the diet provides any health benefits. In fact, it may lead to nutrient deficiencies if not done carefully.

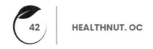

FREQUENTLY ASKED QUESTIONS

8. Is the keto diet safe for long-term use?
The keto diet, which is very low in carbohydrates and high in fats, can be effective for short-term weight loss, but its long-term safety is still debated. Some individuals may experience nutrient deficiencies, digestive issues, or elevated cholesterol levels when on keto for an extended period. It's important to ensure you're still getting adequate fiber, vitamins, and minerals. Consulting a healthcare provider before starting any long-term restrictive diet is advisable.

9. How many meals a day should I eat?
The number of meals you should eat in a day can vary depending on individual preferences, lifestyle factors, and dietary goals. While some people may thrive on three meals a day, others may prefer smaller, more frequent meals or intermittent fasting patterns. Ultimately, it's essential to listen to your body's hunger cues and honor your unique dietary requirements. The key is to focus on balanced, nutrient-rich meals that provide sustained energy and support overall health and well-being, regardless of the specific number of meals consumed each day.

10. Is eating late at night bad for weight management?
The timing of your meals is less important than the overall quality and quantity of your diet. Eating late at night won't necessarily cause weight gain unless it leads to overeating or choosing unhealthy foods. If you're hungry at night, opt for lighter, nutrient-dense snacks, such as fruits, vegetables, or yogurt, and focus on your overall daily intake rather than the time of day.

11. Are all fats bad for you?
No, not all fats are bad. Unsaturated fats, found in foods like avocados, nuts, and olive oil, are actually beneficial for heart health when consumed in moderation. It's saturated and trans fats, found in processed foods and fried foods, that should be limited. Focus on incorporating healthy fats such as avocados, nuts, seeds, olive oil, and fatty fish. These provide essential fatty acids and help with nutrient absorption. It's more about moderating portion sizes than cutting out fats entirely.

12. Should I avoid carbohydrates to lose weight?
Carbohydrates are an essential energy source, especially for the brain and muscles; they should not be completely avoided. Instead, focus on consuming complex carbohydrates like whole grains, fruits, and vegetables which provides sustained energy and fiber. Moderating intake of refined carbohydrates like white bread and sugary snacks can spike blood sugar and provide little nutritional benefit.

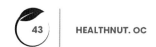

FOUNDATIONS OF NUTRITION

13. How much protein do I really need?
Protein needs vary depending on factors like age, activity level, and fitness goals. For most adults, a general guideline is 0.8-1.0 grams of protein per kilogram of body weight. Athletes or those looking to build muscle may need more, around 1.2-2.0 grams per kilogram.

It's important to spread your protein intake evenly throughout the day—rather than consuming large amounts in one meal—because your body can only use a certain amount of protein at a time for muscle protein synthesis (building and repairing muscles). Spacing it out helps to keep protein synthesis active throughout the day, supporting muscle recovery, repair, and growth more effectively. Excess protein not used for these processes is either stored as fat or excreted, and won't necessarily lead to additional muscle gain.

14. How can I make healthier food choices when eating out?
When eating out, look for options that include plenty of vegetables, lean proteins, and whole grains to reflect MyPlate as explained in the Portion Sizes section. Opt for grilled, steamed, or baked dishes instead of fried foods, and watch portion sizes. You can also ask for sauces and dressings on the side to control your intake of added fats and sugars.

15. Is it necessary to take dietary supplements?
For most people with a balanced diet, dietary supplements are not necessary. However, certain populations, such as pregnant women, older adults, and individuals with specific medical conditions, may benefit from supplementation under the guidance of a healthcare professional.

16. What role do supplements play in enhancing sports performance?
While some supplements may have a modest impact on sports performance, they should be used judiciously and in conjunction with a balanced diet. A couple supplements to consider to optimize performance and support recovery include collagen for joint health or omega-3 for muscle recovery. Many claims about performance-enhancing supplements are exaggerated, and some may even be harmful. It's always best to consult with a healthcare professional or registered dietitian before incorporating supplements into your regimen to ensure they align with your individual needs and goals.

TABLE OF
CONTENTS

FOUNDATIONS OF NUTRITION
EXTRA GOODS
{ APPENDIX }

ENDING NOTE

THANK YOU! for taking the time to read "Foundations of Nutrition" I hope it has provided you with valuable insights and guidance on your nutritional journey. Your commitment to learning and improving your health is truly commendable. For continued support, fresh ideas, and ongoing encouragement, follow me on Instagram and Facebook @healthnut.oc!

In addition to the information provided in the book, I've included several handouts in the "Extra Goods" (Appendix) section to further support your efforts. These resources are designed to be practical tools that you can easily incorporate into your daily routine. Here's how you can utilize them:

1. **Blank Grocery Shopping List**: Didn't have time to plan your meals for the week? Don't fret! Take this shopping list the next time you go to the grocery store, and you'll have all the essentials you need without the stress of last-minute planning.

2. **Meal Planning Sheet**: Use this sheet to plan your days down to the hour, along with your meals for the week. It's a comprehensive tool to keep track of your to-do lists, hydration, mood, sleep, and goals. This sheet will help you stay organized and focused on your health objectives.

3. **Strategic Snacking**: Find options for food products within each MyPlate category, along with their calorie and protein content. This section provides examples of strategic snack options to help with satiety between meals, depending on your weight management goals.

4. **Dining Out at Restaurants**: Your social life shouldn't deter you from your nutrition goals! This handout offers tips on how to order at restaurants so you can continue working towards your goals. It includes "choose this vs. that" options to help you decipher the menu and make nutrient-dense choices while dining out. However, still make room for the soul nourishing foods too!

5. **Lifestyle Feeding Example**: This practical example shows demonstrates how these strategies can fit seamlessly into your daily routine, helping you achieve your nutrition and health goals.

These handouts are designed to be your companions on your journey to enhance your ability to maintain a balanced and nutritious diet, no matter your lifestyle or schedule. Use them to stay organized, make informed choices, and maintain a balanced, healthy lifestyle. Thank you again for reading, and I wish you the best on your adventure towards enhanced wellness!

BLANK GROCERY LIST

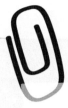

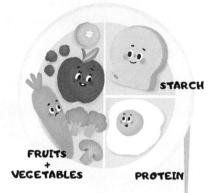

FRUITS + VEGETABLES

STARCH

PROTEIN

FOR WHEN YOU CAN'T PLAN MEALS

3 **VEGGIES** - MEALS, LEAFY GREEN, SNACKING

3 **PROTEINS** - MEATLESS, FISH, MEAT

2 **GRAINS** - BREAKFAST AND DINNER

2 **FRUITS** - SNACKING AND MEALS

2 **DIPS / SPREADS** - VEGGIES AND FRUITS

BLANK GROCERY LIST

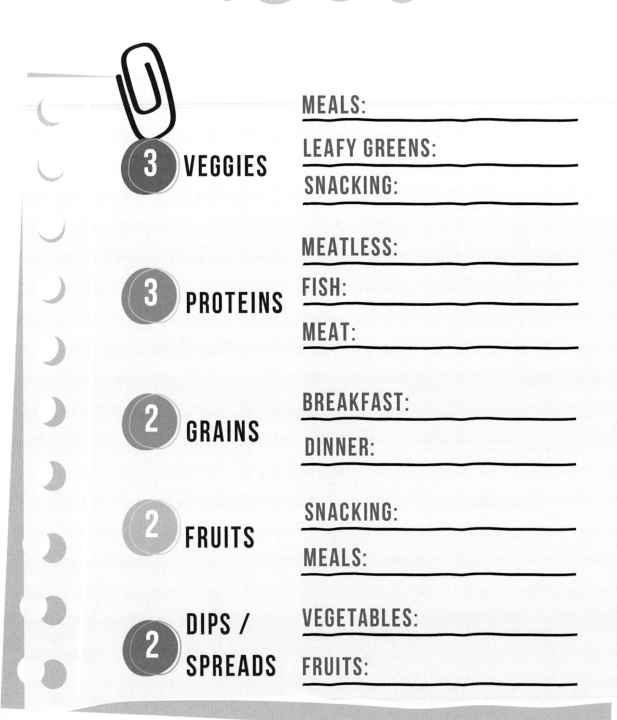

3 VEGGIES

MEALS: _____

LEAFY GREENS: _____

SNACKING: _____

3 PROTEINS

MEATLESS: _____

FISH: _____

MEAT: _____

2 GRAINS

BREAKFAST: _____

DINNER: _____

2 FRUITS

SNACKING: _____

MEALS: _____

2 DIPS / SPREADS

VEGETABLES: _____

FRUITS: _____

DAILY SCHEDULE

TODAY'S DATE: _____   S M T W T F S

MOOD:

ANGRY   TIRED   SAD   GREAT   FUN

☐ _____ 6AM

_____

☐ _____ 8AM

_____

☐ _____ 10AM

_____

☐ _____ 12PM

_____

☐ _____ 2PM

_____

☐ _____ 4PM

_____

☐ _____ 6PM

_____

☐ _____ 8PM

_____

☐ _____ 10PM

_____

WATER INTAKE: (8 oz Glasses)

TODAY'S GOAL:

_____

_____

HOURS OF SLEEP: (Hours)

🌙 🌙 🌙 🌙 🌙 🌙 🌙 🌙

1   2   3   4   5   6   7   8

TO DO:

_____ ☐

_____ ☐

_____ ☐

_____ ☐

_____ ☐

_____ ☐

BREAKFAST:

_____

_____

LUNCH:

_____

_____

DINNER:

_____

_____

DAILY SCHEDULE

TODAY'S DATE: _____   S M T W T F S

MOOD:

ANGRY   TIRED   SAD   GREAT   FUN

☐ _____ 6AM

☐ _____ 8AM

☐ _____ 10AM

☐ _____ 12PM

☐ _____ 2PM

☐ _____ 4PM

☐ _____ 6PM

☐ _____ 8PM

☐ _____ 10PM

WATER INTAKE: (8 oz Glasses)

TODAY'S GOAL:

_____

_____

HOURS OF SLEEP: (Hours)

🌙 🌙 🌙 🌙 🌙 🌙 🌙 🌙
1   2   3   4   5   6   7   8

TO DO:

_____ ☐
_____ ☐
_____ ☐
_____ ☐
_____ ☐
_____ ☐

BREAKFAST:

_____

_____

LUNCH:

_____

_____

DINNER:

_____

STRATEGIC SNACKING

Welcome to your guide on Strategic Snacking – a comprehensive approach to optimizing snacking habits for improved health. Smart snacking goes beyond mere indulgence; it's about **making informed choices that fuel your body efficiently**. In this handout, we delve into the concept of strategic snacking, which involves the art of combining two food groups together to create satisfying and nourishing snacks.

While the nutrition information provided here is an estimation, it's essential to note that actual amounts may vary slightly by brand. For personalized guidance on choosing the best snack options to meet your specific nutrition goals, consult with your registered dietitian nutritionist (RDN). Let's embark on this journey of strategic snacking together, to nourish your body and fuel your life.

Milk and Dairy			
Foods	**Serving Size**	**Calories**	**Protein (g)**
Skim Milk	1 Cup	134	10.3
Nonfat Milk	1 Cup	93	9.3
Soy Milk	1 Cup	105	6
String Cheese	1 Ounce	81	7.1
Cottage Cheese	1/2 Cup	120	13
Greek Yogurt (non-fat, plain)	5.3 oz	80	14.7
Kefir (low-fat, plain)	1 Cup	110	10

STRATEGIC SNACKING

Protein			
Foods	Serving Size	Calories	Protein (g)
Meat (beef, pork, chicken, turkey, fish)	1 Ounce	55 to 100	7
Egg	1 Egg	75	6
Nut Butters (peanut or almond)	2 tablespoons	190	8
Nuts and Seeds	1 Ounce	160 to 200	4 to 6
Bean, Peas, and Lentils	1/2 Cup	100 to 120	14 to 18
Hummus	1/4 Cup	120	6
Tofu	1/2 Cup	100	10
Peanut Buttter	2 tablespoon	60	6

STRATEGIC SNACKING

Grains			
aim for whole grain variations to increase fiber intake			
Foods	Serving Size	Calories	Protein (g)
Bread, Muffins	varies	varies	varies
Pasta, Rice, and Quinoa	varies	varies	varies
Granola, Cereals	varies	varies	varies

Vegetables			
For weight loss + maintenance: Any with added protein dip	varies	varies	varies
For weight gain: Any with fat dip or dressing	varies	varies	varies

Fruit			
Any Fruit	varies	varies	varies
Dried Fruit (ex. raisins, or figs)	2 ounces	160 to 185	0

STRATEGIC SNACKING

*Other			
Foods	**Serving Size**	**Calories**	**Protein (g)**
Avocado	1/2 avocado	100 to 150	2
Cream Cheese	1 tablespoon	50	
Dips	varies	varies	varies
Olives	10 olives	50	0
Salad Dressing	1 tablespoon	50	0
Sour Cream	1 tablespoon	30	0
Canned Coconut Milk	1 tablespoon	25	0

*Fats + Oils			
Sugar, Honey, Jam, Jelly, or Syrup	1 tablespoon	50	0
Gravy	4 tablespoon	25	1

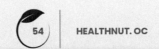

STRATEGIC SNACKING

Supplements			
Meal Replacement Bar	1 Bar	150 to 250	5 o 15
High Kcal, High Protein Drink	1 Drink	200 to 350	10 to 20
Protein Powder (unflavored)	1 tablespoon	25	6

*In categories (Fats + Oils, and Other), it's crucial to be mindful of serving sizes — especially for individuals aiming to maintain or lose weight. These options can be calorie-dense, and even a small amount can significantly contribute to your daily intake.

Remember, moderation is key, and a little goes a long way in supporting your health goals.

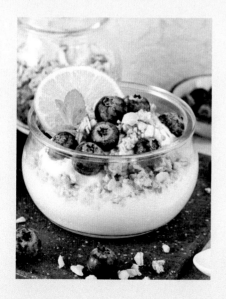
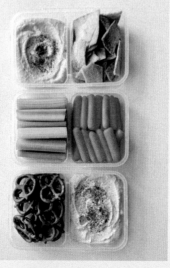
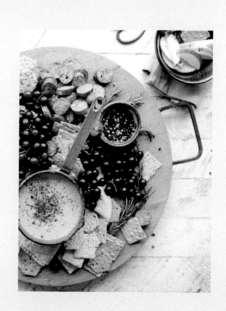

NUTRITIOUS SNACKS
ON - THE - GO

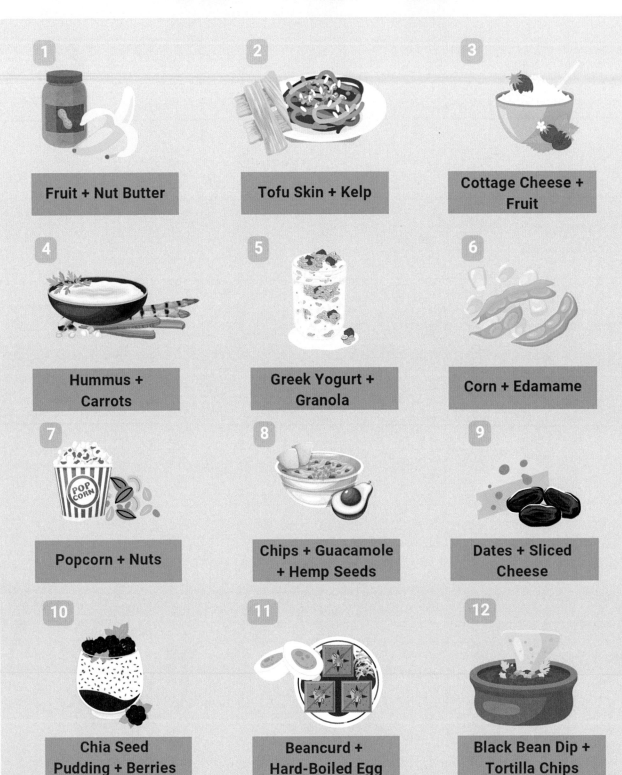

1. Fruit + Nut Butter

2. Tofu Skin + Kelp

3. Cottage Cheese + Fruit

4. Hummus + Carrots

5. Greek Yogurt + Granola

6. Corn + Edamame

7. Popcorn + Nuts

8. Chips + Guacamole + Hemp Seeds

9. Dates + Sliced Cheese

10. Chia Seed Pudding + Berries

11. Beancurd + Hard-Boiled Egg

12. Black Bean Dip + Tortilla Chips

SMART SNACKING

Whether your goal is weight loss, maintenance, or gain, we have tailored calorie targets to suit your needs – **100 calories for weight loss, 200 calories for weight maintenance, and 250+ calories for weight gain.** Additionally, regardless of your weight goals, aiming for **10-15 grams of protein per snack** ensures sustained energy and satiety.

100 calories (weight loss friendly)

- Edamame (1/2 cup) + 1 tbsp olive oil
- Hummus (1/4 cup) with vegetables
- Tortilla chips + salsa + 2 tbsp sour cream OR 1/2 cup bean dip
- Roasted chickpeas (1/4 cup) + salt & pepper
- Chai latte made with soy milk
- Frozen waffle with 1 tbsp nut butter
- English muffin + 1 egg
- Chia seed pudding (1/4 cup) + blueberries
- Scrambled egg with 1/4 avocado
- Trail mix (1/4 cup)
- Cottage cheese (1/2 cup) + sliced peaches
- Baked tofu (1/2 cup) with dip
- Hot chocolate made with nonfat/skim milk
- Smoothie made with 1 cup Kefir + strawberries

200 calories (weight maintenance)

- Greek yogurt (1/2 cup) chopped nuts/seeds/dried fruit/chia seeds or flax seeds)
- Rice or pasta (1/2 cup) with 1 tbsp olive oil + 1 tbsp Parmesan cheese
- English muffin + 1 tbsp nut butter
- Sliced apple/banana or 1 ounce of pretzels with 2 tbsp nut butter
- Plain bagel + 2 tbsp cream cheese
- 2 graham crackers + turkey slice (1 oz) + string cheese cheese
- Lunchmeat + cheese roll ups (2)
- Nut butter and jelly sandwich
- Hummus (1/4 cup) with pita bread
- Trail mix (1/4 cup) with popcorn
- 4 soup dumplings + steamed vegetables
- Zucchini bread slice + nut butter

SMART SNACKING

More than 250 calories (weight gain)

- Chicken, tuna, or egg salad (1/2 cup) on bread or crackers + 1 cup milk
- Milkshake made with 2 tbsp nut butter, 1 frozen banana, 1/2 cup whole milk, 1/2 cup ice cream
- Chicken drumstick and 1/2 cup mashed potatoes
- Oatmeal (1 cup) cooked with 1/2 cup milk, 1 tbsp brown sugar and 1 tbsp raisin
- Ice cream (1/2 cup) topped with 1 ounce chopped nuts
- Snack wrap: 1 corn tortilla, 2 slices ham, 2 slices cheese, 1 tbsp mayonnaise
- Stuffed pita: 1/4 cup hummus, sliced avocado, olives, tomatoes
- 1 grilled cheese or quesadilla

Other Ideas:

_____

_____

_____

_____

_____

_____

_____

_____

_____

DINING OUT AT RESTAURANTS

What if I said you can **enjoy your social life while maintaining your health goals**? The following offers practical advice on how to navigate dining out while staying true to your wellness objectives. Recall the principles of MyPlate discussed in section 2. When making choices at restaurants, **opt for dishes that are nutrient-dense while minimizing added sugars, saturated fat, and sodium**. Start with these tips:

01 Decode the Menu

- Look for choices that are **baked, broiled, grilled, poached, steamed, boiled, or roasted** to limit extra saturated fat and salt.
- If unsure, ask your server how menu items are prepared and/or if they can be prepared a different way.

02 Add Color!

- Choose dishes that **incorporate plenty of color** (fruits and vegetables) whether as main entrees or side dishes.
- If you **start your meal with vegetables or salad first**, you will feel full sooner and ensure that you are getting fiber, vitamins, and minerals.

03 Select Lean Protein

- Choose lean protein options such as **chicken, fish, tofu, beans, or legumes**. As mentioned above, check to see how menu items are prepared.
- These choices are lower in saturated fat and provide essential amino acids necessary for muscle repair and overall body function.

04 Split Your Dish

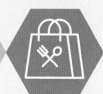

Food portions at restaurants are often very large:
- Consider **sharing a meal** with a dining companion or ask for a **half portion**.
- **Request a to-go box** at the beginning of the meal and set aside a portion of your meal to enjoy at your next meal

05 Choose Your Sauce

- **Pick sauces made from vegetables** like marinara vs cream or butter sauces to limit calories from saturated fat.
- Ask your server for **sauces on the side** or to prepare the dish with **less sauce or no sauce.**

Final Tips!

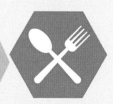

Dining out should be an enjoyable experience. Enjoying the occasional dessert will not derail your progress. Instead of fixating on restrictions, focus on incorporating nutritious foods into your meal. **Approach dining out as a give-and-take situation**, where you make informed choices that align with your health objectives while still allowing yourself to enjoy the moment.

INSTEAD OF THIS		CHOOSE THIS
* fried chicken * meat lover pizza * deep-fried fish * butter, gravy, cream-based sauces	MAIN DISHES	* rotisserie-style chicken (skin removed) * meat pizza with vegetable toppings * grilled, steamed, or baked fish * vegetable-based sauces
* mayonnaise, tartar sauce, special sauce * bacon, pork, roast beef * chicken / tuna salad * breaded chicken * deluxe hamburger	SANDWICHES HAMBURGERS	* mustard or low-fat mayonnaise * lean meats (chicken, turkey) * add vegetables to sandwich or side salad * grilled chicken * plain hamburger
* large french fries * cheese and sour cream * Italian, Caesar, blue cheese, ranch dressing * onion rings, mozzarella sticks, french fries	SIDE DISHES	* share small french fries * low-fat cheese and sour cream * vinaigrette dressing; ask that it be served on the side, and use less * order vegetables or salad
* soft-drink or milkshake * cakes, cookies, pies	BEVERAGES DESSERTS	* water, 100% fruit juice, unsweetened iced tea, fat-free/low-fat milk * small or sugar-free soft drink * small dessert, fat-free frozen yogurt, low-fat ice cream, sherbet

GROCERY LIST EXAMPLE

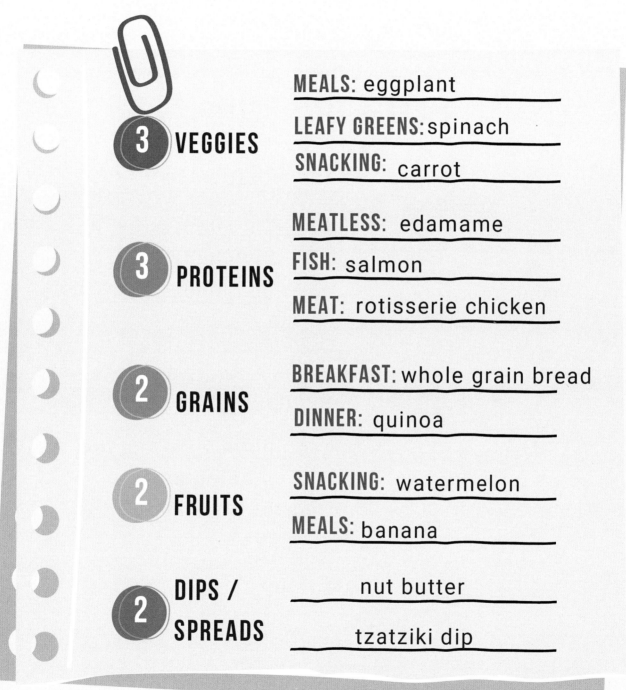

3 VEGGIES
- MEALS: eggplant
- LEAFY GREENS: spinach
- SNACKING: carrot

3 PROTEINS
- MEATLESS: edamame
- FISH: salmon
- MEAT: rotisserie chicken

2 GRAINS
- BREAKFAST: whole grain bread
- DINNER: quinoa

2 FRUITS
- SNACKING: watermelon
- MEALS: banana

2 DIPS / SPREADS
- nut butter
- tzatziki dip

GROCERY LIST
MEAL EXAMPLES

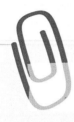

INGREDIENTS TO MEALS

BREAKFAST

banana nut butter toast

salmon tzatziki toast with edamame

LUNCH

chicken quinoa bowl

salmon salad toast

DINNER

eggplant quinoa bowl

salmon plate with roasted vegetables

SNACKS

carrot tzatziki dip

watermelon banana smoothie with nut butter

DAILY SCHEDULE

TODAY'S DATE: *EXAMPLE DAY 1*

S M T W T F S

MOOD: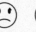

ANGRY TIRED SAD GREAT FUN

☐	WAKE UP	6AM
	BREAKFAST	
☐		8AM
☐	MORNING SNACK:	10AM

WATERMELON BANANA NUT BUTTER SMOOTHIE
(178 KCALS, 9 G PRO, 21 G CARBS, 7 G FAT)

☐		12PM
	LUNCH	
☐		2PM
☐	AFTERNOON SNACK:	4PM

BANANA
(105 KCALS, 1 G PRO, 24 G CARBS, 0.4 G FAT)

WORKOUT

☐	DINNER	6PM
☐	EVENING SNACK:	8PM

CARROTS W/ TZATZIKI DIP + EDAMAME
(134 KCALS, 10 G PRO, 7 G CARBS, 5 G FAT)

☐	BEDTIME	10PM

WATER INTAKE: (8 oz Glasses)

💧 💧 💧 💧 💧 💧 💧

TODAY'S GOAL:

_____

_____

HOURS OF SLEEP: (Hours)

🌙 🌙 🌙 🌙 🌙 🌙 🌙 🌙
1   2   3   4   5   6   7   8

TO DO:

_____ ☐
_____ ☐
_____ ☐
_____ ☐
_____ ☐
_____ ☐

BREAKFAST:
(404 KCALS, 40 G PRO, 18 G CARBS, 17 G FAT)
1 WHOLE WHEAT TOAST W/ 3 OZ SALMON +
TZATZIKI SAUCE + EDAMAME + 8 OZ SOY MILK

LUNCH:
(500 KCALS, 35 G PRO, 36 G CARBS, 21 G FAT)
1 CUP QUINOA BOWL W/ 3 OZ CHICKEN,
1 CUP SPINACH, BALSAMIC VINEGAR + OLIVE OIL

DINNER:
(470 KCALS, 32 G PRO, 41 G CARBS, 16 G FAT)
MEDITERRANEAN SALMON TZATZIKI BOWL W/
1 CUP QUINOA BOWL + 1 CUP ROASTED VEGETABLES

DAILY SCHEDULE

TODAY'S DATE: 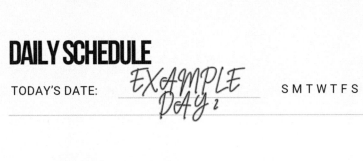 EXAMPLE DAY 2

S M T W T F S

MOOD:

ANGRY   TIRED   SAD   GREAT   FUN

- [ ] **WAKE UP**   6AM
  MORNING SNACK:
      WATERMELON
  (29 KCALS, 1 G PRO, 7 G CARBS, 0.1 G FAT)

- [ ] **WORKOUT**   8AM

  BREAKFAST

- [ ]   10AM

- [ ] **LUNCH**   12PM

- [ ]   2PM

  AFTERNOON SNACK:
      NUT BUTTER BANANA SMOOTHIE
  (155 KCALS, 20 G PRO, 17 G CARBS, 1 G FAT)
- [ ]   4PM

- [ ] **DINNER**   6PM

- [ ] **EVENING SNACK:**   8PM
  CARROTS W/ TZATZIKI DIP + EDAMAME
  (134 KCALS, 10 G PRO, 7 G CARBS, 5 G FAT)

- [ ] **BEDTIME**   10PM

WATER INTAKE: (8 oz Glasses)

💧💧💧💧💧💧💧

TODAY'S GOAL:

HOURS OF SLEEP: (Hours)

🌙 🌙 🌙 🌙 🌙 🌙 🌙 🌙
1   2   3   4   5   6   7   8

TO DO:

- [ ]
- [ ]
- [ ]
- [ ]
- [ ]
- [ ]

BREAKFAST:
(430 KCALS, 22 G PRO, 42 G CARBS, 18 G FAT)
    1 WHOLE WHEAT TOAST W/ BANANA +

    2 TBSP NUT BUTTER + 8 OZ SOY MILK

LUNCH:
(590 KCALS, 38 G PRO, 41 G CARBS, 26 G FAT)
    3 OZ SALMON SALAD TOAST W/ SPINACH +

    MASHED EDAMAME + TZATZIKI SAUCE

DINNER:
(510 KCALS, 22 G PRO, 81 G CARBS, 7 G FAT)
    THAI QUINOA BOWL W/ 1/2 CUP EDAMAME +

    1 CUP SPINACH + CARROTS + NUT BUTTER SAUCE

DAILY SCHEDULE

TODAY'S DATE: *EXAMPLE DAY 3*   S M T W T F S

MOOD:
ANGRY   TIRED   SAD   GREAT   FUN

☐ **WAKE UP**   6AM

  BREAKFAST

☐   8AM
_____

☐ **MORNING SNACK:**   10AM
ROASTED VEGGIES WITH TZATZIKI SAUCE + EDAMAME
(230 KCALS, 10 G PRO, 17 G CARBS, 5 G FAT)
_____

☐ **LUNCH**   12PM

_____

☐   2PM
_____

☐ **AFTERNOON SNACK:**
        BANANA   4PM
(105 KCALS, 1 G PRO, 24 G CARBS, 0.4 G FAT)

☐ **WORKOUT**   6PM

_____

☐ **DINNER**   8PM

_____

☐ **BEDTIME**   10PM

WATER INTAKE: (8 oz Glasses)

💧 💧 💧 💧 💧 💧 💧

TODAY'S GOAL:
_____
_____

HOURS OF SLEEP: (Hours)

🌙 🌙 🌙 🌙 🌙 🌙 🌙 🌙
1   2   3   4   5   6   7   8

TO DO:
_____ ☐
_____ ☐
_____ ☐
_____ ☐
_____ ☐
_____ ☐

BREAKFAST:
(409 KCALS, 40 G PRO, 27 G CARBS, 16 G FAT)
1 WHOLE WHEAT TOAST W/ 3 OZ SALMON +
TZATZIKI SAUCE + SPINACH + 8 OZ SOY MILK

LUNCH:
(500 KCALS, 31 G PRO, 29 G CARBS, 25 G FAT)
1/2 CUP QUINOA SALAD W/ 3 OZ CHICKEN,
1 CUP SPINACH, 1/2 CUP CARROTS, TZATZIKI SAUCE

DINNER:
(421 KCALS, 37 G PRO, 37 G CARBS, 14 G FAT)
3 OZ GRILLED SALMON BOWL W/ 1/2 CUP
QUINOA, 1 CUP ROASTED EGGPLANT + EDAMAME

REFERENCES

1. Albosta M, Bakke J. Intermittent fasting: is there a role in the treatment of diabetes A review of the literature and guide for primary care physicians. Clin Diabetes Endocrinol. 2021;7(1):3. Published 2021 Feb 3. doi:10.1186/s40842-020-00116-1

2. All Your Hand Portion Questions, Answered. Precision Nutrition. Published April 12, 2021. https://www.precisionnutrition.com/hand-portion-faq

3. Calcagno M, Kahleova H, Alwarith J, et al. The Thermic Effect of Food: A Review. J Am Coll Nutr. 2019;38(6):547-551. doi:10.1080/07315724.2018.1552544

4. Dine Out / Take Out | MyPlate. www.myplate.gov. https://www.myplate.gov/tip-sheet/dine-out-take-out

5. DiNicolantonio JJ, O'Keefe J. The Importance of Maintaining a Low Omega-6/Omega-3 Ratio for Reducing the Risk of Autoimmune Diseases, Asthma, and Allergies. Mo Med. 2021;118(5):453-459.

6. Halton TL, Hu FB. The effects of high protein diets on thermogenesis, satiety and weight loss: a critical review. J Am Coll Nutr. 2004;23(5):373-385. doi:10.1080/07315724.2004.10719381

7. Hwangbo DS, Lee HY, Abozaid LS, Min KJ. Mechanisms of Lifespan Regulation by Calorie Restriction and Intermittent Fasting in Model Organisms. Nutrients. 2020;12(4):1194. Published 2020 Apr 24. doi:10.3390/nu12041194

8. [Infographic] The best calorie control guide. Estimating portion size and food intake just got a whole lot easier. Precision Nutrition. Published December 7, 2016. https://www.precisionnutrition.com/calorie-control-guide-infographic

9. Karpinski C, Rosenbloom C, And N. Sports Nutrition: A Handbook for Professionals. Academy Of Nutrition And Dietetics; 2017.

10. Moris JM, Heinold C, Blades A, Koh Y. Nutrient-Based Appetite Regulation. J Obes Metab Syndr. 2022;31(2):161-168. doi:10.7570/jomes22031

11. Reguant-Closa A, Harris MM, Lohman TG, Meyer NL. Validation of the Athlete's Plate Nutrition Educational Tool: Phase I. Int J Sport Nutr Exerc Metab. 2019;29(6):628-635. doi:10.1123/ijsnem.2018-0346

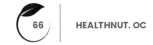

REFERENCES

12. Sareen Gropper. Advanced Nutrition and Human Metabolism. 8th ed. Cengage Learning Custom P; 2021.

13. Reguant-Closa A, Roesch A, Lansche J, Nemecek T, Lohman TG, Meyer NL. The Environmental Impact of the Athlete's Plate Nutrition Education Tool. Nutrients. 2020;12(8):2484. Published 2020 Aug 18. doi:10.3390/nu12082484

13. Roach LA, Woolfe W, Bastian B, Neale EP, Francois ME. Systematic literature review: should a bedtime snack be used to treat hyperglycemia in type 2 diabetes?. Am J Clin Nutr. 2022;116(5):1251-1264. doi:10.1093/ajcn/nqac245

14. Robertson R. Omega-3-6-9 Fatty Acids: A Complete Overview. Healthline. Published 2017. https://www.healthline.com/nutrition/omega-3-6-9-overview

15. Schübel R, Nattenmüller J, Sookthai D, et al. Effects of intermittent and continuous calorie restriction on body weight and metabolism over 50 wk: a randomized controlled trial. Am J Clin Nutr. 2018;108(5):933-945. doi:10.1093/ajcn/nqy196

16. Thomas DT, Erdman KA, Burke LM. American College of Sports Medicine Joint Position Statement. Nutrition and Athletic Performance [published correction appears in Med Sci Sports Exerc. 2017 Jan;49(1):222. doi: 10.1249/MSS.0000000000001162]. Med Sci Sports Exerc. 2016;48(3):543-568. doi:10.1249/MSS.0000000000000852

17. Thomas DT, Erdman KA, Burke LM. Position of the Academy of Nutrition and Dietetics, Dietitians of Canada, and the American College of Sports Medicine: Nutrition and Athletic Performance [published correction appears in J Acad Nutr Diet. 2017 Jan;117(1):146. doi: 10.1016/j.jand.2016.11.008]. J Acad Nutr Diet. 2016;116(3):501-528. doi:10.1016/j.jand.2015.12.006

18. Tips on eating out. Nursing. 2006;36(8):69. doi:https://doi.org/10.1097/00152193-200608000-00050

19. USDA. Dietary Guidelines for Americans 2020 -2025 . USDA; 2020. https://www.dietaryguidelines.gov/sites/default/files/2020-12/Dietary_Guidelines_for_Americans_2020-2025.pdf

20. USDA. What is MyPlate? www.myplate.gov. Published 2020. https://www.myplate.gov/eat-healthy/what-is-myplate

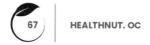

MY NOTES

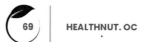

MY NOTES

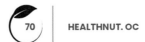

MY NOTES

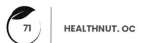

MY NOTES

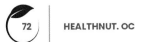

MY NOTES

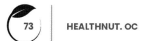

MY NOTES

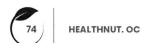

MY NOTES

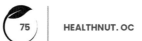

MY NOTES

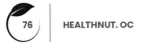

MY NOTES

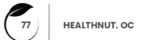

MY NOTES

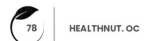

Made in the USA
Las Vegas, NV
02 January 2025

049a8f04-abfe-47e1-b004-46d23d98ab23R01